ARABELLA WEIR
The Real Me is Thin

FOURTH ESTATE · *London*

Fourth Estate
An imprint of HarperCollins*Publishers*
77–85 Fulham Palace Road
Hammersmith
London W6 8JB

This Fourth Estate paperback edition published 2011
1

First published in Great Britain by Fourth Estate in 2010

Copyright © Arabella Weir 2010

Arabella Weir asserts the moral right to
be identified as the author of this work

A catalogue record for this book is available from the British Library

ISBN 978-0-00-738660-4

Set in Adobe Caslon and Futura by Birdy Book Design

Printed and bound in Great Britain by Clays Ltd, St Ives plc

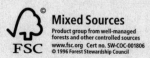

Mixed Sources
Product group from well-managed
forests and other controlled sources
www.fsc.org Cert no. SW-COC-001806
© 1996 Forest Stewardship Council
FSC

FSC is a non-profit international organization established to promote the
responsible management of the world's forests. Products carrying the FSC
label are independently certified to assure consumers that they come
from forests that are managed to meet the social, economic, and
ecological needs of present and future generations

Find out more about HarperCollins and the environment at
www.harpercollins.co.uk/green

All rights reserved. No part of this publication may be reproduced,
stored in a retrieval system, or transmitted, in any form or by any means,
electronic, mechanical, photocopying, recording or otherwise, without
the prior permission of the publishers.

This book is sold subject to the condition that it shall not, by way of trade
or otherwise, be lent, re-sold, hired out or otherwise circulated without the
publisher's prior consent in any form of binding or cover other than that in
which it is published and without a similar condition including this
condition being imposed on the subsequent purchaser.

For Helen Scott-Lidgett,
a very good friend and true inspiration
to all who know her.

EDINBURGH LIBRARIES	
C0044367740	
Bertrams	05/07/2011
	£7.99
CE	RA784

Contents

Preface: how to tell if you think you're fat   ix

The real me is thin   1

When their ship came in   5

Open the box   10

'Arabella's fat'   15

Too much   23

Daddy's girl   32

Happiness is a warm scone   40

Cooking blind   48

Shock in awe   53

Funny valentine   59

My other family   65

A waist of time   71

Kurt Waldheim finds out I'm fat   81

All you can eat at the boy buffet   91

My fairy stepmother   97

This isn't just food . . .   107

Actresses don't eat   114

Doctor No   128

Allergies for attention   135

The appeal of obliteration   142

Everyone's got an opinion   149

Passive-aggressive pudding   156

Flying spaghetti   163

Outing my bum   169

Don't eat pudding if you want to get a job
   (or a boyfriend)   176

Sexual eating   182

The mother of all diets   189

Feeding Mum   197

Dieting makes you fat   203

Not eating, just neatening   208

Wrong thinking   215

Happy ending?   221

Acknowledgements   227

Preface: how to tell if you think you're fat

All women think they're fat – whether they are or not, because all women *feel* fat. Well, here's how to tell if you think you're fat, too.

TEN TOP TIPS

You think you're fat if:

- You're reading this book.

- You think *not* eating is a good thing.

- *You* think you're fat even though no one else does.

- You think you'd like yourself better if you were thinner.

- You think that people who *don't* eat are better than you.

- Unless catering for others, you have nothing in your fridge except a small sliver of mouldy cheese and a rancid piece of fruit, both of which you'd eat rather than chuck out.

- You never order pudding but eat a bit of someone else's.

- You decide not to have a glass of wine because you're 'not drinking at the moment', but then have half a glass (not in a wineglass), and then top it up but only half-way again, and so on – but manage to end your evening still kidding yourself you didn't have a drink.

- You've got clothes in your cupboard that are too small for you and you've never worn but can't chuck out because they *are* going to fit just as soon as you've lost some weight.

- The title of this book means anything to you.

The real me is thin

The real me is thin. Of course she is. The *real* me does not need a size 18 (sometimes even a 20) to accommodate her mammoth arse (not my real one, obviously) when buying trousers. Properly huge women wear sizes 18 and 20, not me. I am not fat. I can't be. I don't feel like a fat woman. Well, not all the time. Obviously, I *feel* like a fat woman a lot of the time. If I didn't, I wouldn't think there was another 'me' out there, another, thin me available somewhere. The fat woman I feel like a lot of the time is my go-to person, the one I feel like when I feel bad about myself, which is how I feel when I eat too much, more often than not, or sometimes eat at all! But that can't be who I *really* am. Admittedly, I find myself temporarily housed in a slightly-larger-than-planned-for body but, you see, that's OK because it's not my real one. You see in my real life – the one I'm supposed to be having, the one I had planned on having, the one I'm going to have – I'll be wearing slinky party dresses with micro spaghetti straps, lovely bikinis and city shorts over patterned tights, of course I will … just as soon as I shake off this fat woman's body, which, as I've pointed out, isn't actually mine anyway. I've no idea who put me into it. I certainly didn't. How could the odd handful of chocolate-covered peanuts, sporadic slices of butter-laden malt loaf, and the occasional bottle of wine in one sitting steadily, over about thirty years, possibly be responsible for getting me into this body? This overweight body I did not plan for and don't recognise?

Right from the beginning – well, my beginning anyway, when I was little – the real me wasn't supposed to be fat. My parents made it clear they did not want a Fat Arabella – they wanted, expected, demanded, even, eventually, a Thin Arabella. The indisputable fact that Thin Arabella had never made an appearance (my birth weight was 11½ pounds) didn't seem to factor into my parents' expectations. They seemed to think that Thin Arabella must be in there somewhere and that I, Fat Arabella, was deliberately hiding her to annoy them. As I grew up it became clear from their confused, slightly irritated reactions whenever I said I was hungry that they didn't know who this girl was. My mum and dad couldn't possibly have been meant to have a Fat Daughter. They'd both got degrees from Oxford, they read important books, spoke foreign languages, played musical instruments – good God, they went to museums for pleasure. People like that don't get fat kids. Other people get fat children, not people who drink real coffee and look down on people who wear driving gloves, go on package tours, and disguise loo rolls under knitted dolls wearing crinolines. My mum and dad were cut out to be winners, and winners' kids aren't fat.

The real me must surely be the one my parents were expecting, the one they had in mind when they longed for a daughter to follow their two boys. When a couple long for a girl they do not long for a fat one. They dream of a sweet, adorable, and, above all else, pretty girl. They must have been mystified. 'Hey, Genepool, we didn't ask for fat! Who ordered the fat one?! Not us!' Who actually wants fat? No one. They certainly didn't dream about having just *any* kind of daughter – thin or fat, ugly or pretty, three legs, four arms . . . They wanted what everyone who yearns for a girl wants: pretty, charming, a little bit cheeky maybe, bright would be a bonus, but not if it's at the cost of being attractive. Winners have gorgeous girls. But what happens when she comes out fat? What then? You still love her, of course you do, you just set about . . . erm . . . modifying her. Encouraging her, shall we say, not to eat; and also perhaps to be a little embarrassed about her body and how much she eats – even if, at the start anyway, she eats only what her siblings eat, yet alarmingly it seems to make her fatter than them. That must be her fault.

So, right from the beginning, the scene was set for a lifetime of believing myself to be fat – whether I was or not. Fat in my head, whatever my body shape. I was a chunky wee thing, and although (I'm told) I was much loved, it felt more like much judged, particularly for my appetite and fluctuating size – a deadly combination, and inextricably linked, according to my parents. If I was hungry it must be because I was greedy, because – seeing as I was evidently not thin – I couldn't ever be genuinely hungry. A message I learnt early on: fat people aren't allowed to be hungry.

Of course, my parents' attitude to my size as I was growing up isn't entirely responsible for my lifelong struggle with food, eating, overeating and weight. I've chosen a number of paths that reinforced my deep-seated belief that Thinner Equals Better; but Mum and Dad's effort to secure themselves a thinner daughter certainly set me off down that road – how could it not?

So here are a few stories from the life of a fat daughter, fat schoolgirl, fat girlfriend, fat actress, fat mum, and fat wife – or, to put it another way, how I got to thinking my bum looked big in everything, whether it did or not.

This book is for any woman or girl trapped in the wrong thinking that there's another, better, 'real' her out there. It's for any woman who has trouble accepting the size and shape she is. Really, it's for any woman who's ever thought twice about anything she's putting into her mouth.

When their ship came in

On 6 December 1957, in an uncharacteristically chilly San Francisco, it snows for the first time in 17 years. A much-longed-for baby girl is born to a British couple living there temporarily. Encouraged by the forward-thinking obstetrician (and very unusually for the time), the father witnesses the birth. A sister for two boys: Andrew, a few weeks away from turning three, and Matthew, a few weeks past turning two. Now the parents have three under three (as they would often say in future years with an air of both pride and disbelief). A telegram – a wild extravagance in those days – dispatched to the parents' parents back in Scotland contains only one word.

Arabella.

That'd be me.

They tell me this story many times over the years. My adored Granny Sheila, my mother's stepmother, also repeats the story many times. It has always made me feel like an important event, like a ship's maiden voyage or a spacecraft successfully circling the sun. No explanation necessary, no further information required. Everyone reading the telegram will understand: that's it, mission accomplished – the longed-for girl has been produced. As the years pass, my mother never fails to add the extra, not so welcome, detail: 'and she weighed nearly 11½ pounds!' So in some ways, given that the average newborn's weight is 7 pounds, I sort of *was* a ship, actually more of a tanker, practically an ocean liner compared to the tiny dinghies most babies are.

The family was in San Francisco awaiting removal to Washington, DC, where my father was to start work at the British Embassy a few months after I was born. I have very few, fragmented recollections of the following four years, except of time spent with our wonderful Jamaican cook and nanny, Innes. She was a short, round, squishy woman who showered us with affection all day long. She wasn't officially our nanny. A fierce Scottish woman had been brought with us to do that job, but she'd soon left, not able to compete with the loving and beloved Innes. Innes used to feed us in front of the television and give us Coca-Cola in glass bottles! A combination of thrilling indulgences tolerated by our parents, thanks to Innes' irresistible charm and easy-going nature.

My parents' marriage was probably at its happiest in Washington. And why wouldn't it have been? Those were the Kennedy years, the Camelot years. Washington was full of exciting, young, politically active people. Professionally, Dad, though still very lowly, was right in the thick of it; Mum got to know other like-minded, bright, capable women and *she didn't have to cook*. What could have been better? Although, unusually for the time, Mum had lived independently before getting married (and had therefore, presumably, fed herself), she'd managed to overlook the obligatory grind that was central to a successful married life – the provision of endless, appetising, not to mention nourishing, meals for children and spouse. It's the iceberg lurking under seemingly calm waters, the unspoken yet taken-for-granted clause of most marriage contracts: there will be cooking, day in, day out, whether you feel like it or not, for year after year after year. In the early Fifties, when my parents married, this chore fell exclusively to women. And there was no discussion about it being a chore. More than 50 years on, little has changed. Sure, there are plenty of flamboyant male cooks around now, taking the sting out of cooking being a 'girly' thing to do, but the relentless daily grind of actually feeding a family still falls to the mother in the vast majority of instances.

In my mother's case, I guess she'd imagined (as she often did about anything that irked her) that if she ignored this inexorable chore, it would somehow go away. Up until that time, though, she hadn't had to deal too much with that most wearing of responsibilities, since they'd had only a few years of married life in London before being posted abroad – and a foreign posting always included an allowance for 'staff'. Obviously, the poorer the country of your posting the more staff you could get, since you were paying wages at the local rate. So, in America in the Fifties as a First Secretary to the British Embassy in Washington, Dad's staff allowance meant they could afford Innes, who was doing the job of both cook and nanny. I'm not sure how many of the changes promised by the burgeoning civil rights movement Innes was ever going to see, but she was much loved and greatly treasured by all our family, even Mum and Dad.

If they were having a big dinner or a party Mum and Innes would cook together. One of the very few positive food-related memories I have of Mum is the sensational sweet-sour salad dressing she made with a 'secret ingredient' she attributed to Innes – dark brown sugar. The dressing was richly brown and gooey, like very liquidy tar, and tasted *so* good. Nowadays, of course, anyone who fancies themselves as a bit of a turn in the kitchen uses sugar in salad dressing, or balsamic vinegar which, tasty as it is, is really just sugar in a bottle. Back then, it was Innes's own invention, or at least a trick brought with her from Jamaica, and I can't taste or make that dressing without thinking of our cuddly, uninhibitedly affectionate nanny-cook.

Mum was a good cook but lazy or rather unconventional about how and when to cook. Added to that she was breezily capricious about meting out food, constantly, and always on a whim, changing her mind about who deserved what. It was like being fed by King Lear. She cared greatly about good-quality food; just not if she was the one who had to provide it. But I can still remember some fantastic things she cooked: chocolate soufflés she'd unintentionally leave in the oven too long, so that the top skin crustified a bit and became chewy and nutty, like a brownie; leeks slow-cooked in olive oil, lemon juice, garlic, and brown sugar (again); mushroom risottos; apple crumbles with raisins and cloves, the crumble buttery and crunchy with sugar. And bread. Mum used to make batches of delicious wholemeal bread long before wholemeal was trendy and everything was suddenly supposed to be home-made and not-white.

But all this stopped when she and Dad started breaking up. I say 'started' because, like some unloved old clapped-out car, they let the marriage limp along for years, giving it an occasional kick to see if it could be made to work properly, but then letting it conk out again, not really knowing if either of them cared enough to put the effort into getting the engine restarted. It's hard to make something work if you don't know whether or not you really want it to. The first time I think I realised my parents were in real trouble was when I bit into a slice of Mum's bread and got a mouthful of rock salt. There was so much of it that the skin on my lips puckered up instantly, as if I'd dived into the Dead Sea with my mouth open. Mum hadn't crushed up the salt properly before mixing it in. That's when I knew things were really beginning to fall apart.

Open the box

I started changing shape and gaining weight as they started breaking up. Actually, I'd say, using as evidence the few photographs there are of me from around that time, 1965–6, my body was simply plumping out, maybe in readiness for puberty, or maybe I was just putting on weight. I don't look as though I'd have needed two seats on the bus, but neither could I be described as svelte. As if to accentuate my non-sylph-like self, I'd been given an all-the-rage-at-the-time Beatles-style pudding-bowl haircut. I don't know whose idea that was. I knew who the Beatles were and I liked them well enough, but I was more of a Monkeys' fan. I don't remember yearning for a Beatles' haircut; quite apart from anything else, they were boys. It's hard to imagine a more inappropriate choice for a not terribly pretty, not very confident, chunky nine-year-old girl. Like some awful judgement barometer, as they started arguing more and more, I started getting rounder and rounder. At the same time Mum became more openly and vocally angry about and resentful of her 'wifely' duties, chief amongst which seemed to be cooking.

After we'd returned to Britain in 1963, with my little sister, Christina, born the year before, we set up home in a large flat in central London while Dad looked for a suitable house to buy. Dad was back in the Foreign Office and I can barely remember him being around at all, and Mum clearly wasn't happy. One day, outside 'eating hours', I complained to Mum, 'I'm hungry.' She replied brusquely, 'Fine. It's good for you.' I didn't know what she meant. I had no idea what she was talking about. At that young age I knew nothing about dieting and the process of denying yourself food in order to lose weight. Mum didn't go on to explain the procedure or my apparent need to know about such things. However, I did immediately realise that my telling her I was hungry had made her cross. And I remember quickly thinking I'd have to get something to eat without her finding out.

There must have been other 'ticking off' incidents related to my hunger and or food before this, but it's the one that sticks in my mind as the moment when the dreaded box was first opened: the box marked 'how to have a neurotic relationship with food' or, depending on who's responsible for producing the box in the first place, you might call it the 'how to give your child an unhealthy attitude to food' box. Or put simply, and without apportioning any blame, it was a key lesson in 'how to get fat'.

Thwarted and confused, I was – naturally – still hungry, and could not begin to work out how the gnawing in my stomach was in any way 'good for me'. Satisfied that I was going to accept her reaction to my announcement, Mum went off while I hung around in the hall. I allowed a few minutes to pass and then strolled casually, with as best a nothing-to-see-here-I'm-not-thinking-about-food-anymore-at-all air as I could fashion, past the open door to the living room, where my mother was now immersed in a book, and snuck into the kitchen.

Once there, I did something I'd never done before and it surprised me. After a last-minute perimeter check I went over to the cupboard, sneaked out a packet of biscuits, and wolfed down the entire thing. As each successive one made its dry, crumbly way down my throat I quickly realised that I didn't actually want the whole packet at all. I knew I only really wanted one or two, but I was panicking by now. It had been made clear that I wasn't going to get any through the approved channels, so I thought I'd better secure as many as I could covertly, and by any means necessary. I was anxious that, when official 'biscuit time' came round, my hunger, left unsated, would be so massive that there simply wouldn't be enough biscuits in the world, never mind in our flat, to hold it at bay. In any case, the prevailing 'biscuit law' in our house meant that no one was ever really allowed more than two for fear of unleashing an avalanche of eyebrow raising and sharp inhalation of breath, accompanied by a tirade of unfavourable comments about what wanting more than two said about your entire personality, and that's leaving aside the very real possibility of being called a 'greedy pig' in front of everyone else.

But to me this hunger wasn't my friend, it wasn't being nice to me, so how could it possibly be 'good for me'? When has hunger ever helped anyone do anything? I was completely bemused. It wasn't like brushing my teeth, which I was always being nagged to do. It was tedious but did at least feel good after I'd done it and I believed it stopped my teeth from falling out. An unfed hunger is a monster on your back. And when you're a hungry child, unable to cater for yourself and someone, apparently deliberately, won't feed you, you just feel upset, enraged, and powerless. From then on the whole 'hunger is good for you, eating is bad for you' became established as a recurring theme in my life and I very quickly lost all sense of proportion regarding food. I lost the ability to distinguish between nice food and food I didn't fancy. I lost the ability to eat moderately. I lost the capacity to know what 'full' meant. I just had to eat what I could when I could. I began to crave food, in any form, all the time.

On that particular biscuit day something had to be done to kill my hunger, and if Mum thought it was so 'good for me' to be hungry, then obviously she wasn't about to help me tackle it to the ground. I couldn't waste time thinking about how many biscuits I actually wanted. Now that I had in my grasp the means of reducing my hunger I just had to stuff in as many as possible before I was discovered. Only that way would I get rid of the hunger, ensure it didn't return soon, and, most importantly, avoid being at the mercy of Mum's erratic feeding regime again that day.

In adult life I've learnt that this kind of bingeing is known as 'ensuring your supply', where you (or more specifically me) do something irrational like, say, cramming down a whole loaf of bread in one go because you fear you won't be allowed any, even a perfectly reasonable slice or two, when the time for eating bread comes along. I'm told that, when a social event is looming, alcoholics who are acknowledged as such by family and friends drink in advance and in secret, downing much more than they need to reach the inebriated state they crave, because they know they can't have one or two drinks in public like everyone else, since that will inevitably lead to questions about their drinking.

My mum and dad, by this time at loggerheads on practically everything, were at least united in the shared worry that their first-born daughter was getting fat and agreed I needed to be reigned in. Once my parents started focusing on my size it was made clear that I wouldn't be allowed to eat the same things my siblings were eating, since they weren't deemed overweight. The scene was now set for what turned out to be a lifetime of feeling under attack by the enemy – hunger, which raged seemingly constantly on one side, with parental disapproval looming on the other. As a result I have never felt entitled to eat nor, moreover, to enjoy eating. Good girls don't eat.

It's probably fair to say that I have never, ever put anything in my mouth without thinking about whether it'll make me fat – well, fatter – and I do mean not one single thing.

'Arabella's fat'

In my experience most family members have affectionate nicknames for each other (or supposedly affectionate, at any rate). If not actual nicknames then a shorthand way of referring to their relatives. These monikers are often taken from a dominant characteristic that particular family member is seen to demonstrate. When we hear people say 'My sister's the bossy one' or 'My brother's the grumpy one', we don't think that's the only trait their sibling has. We know what they're talking about. We understand that it's their 'thing' and that that person is more neat or bossy than the rest of his/her family. We are 'placed' by our family members and our position is carved out from early on. It doesn't have to mean very much at all about how your family gets along. It's just something families do, bigger ones especially. The same is true of school friends and work colleagues; any group of people spending a lot of time together replicate a family of some sort.

Your position in your own family may be perfectly benign and extend to no more than being 'the forgetful one' or 'the tidy one'. However, if the label your family gives you is reductive, and informs how they treat you, then it's less benign and harder to break away from. In my family, for blindingly obvious reasons (not least because it was said out loud), I was the fat one. Even when I'd grown up and sometimes wasn't actually fat (or, rather, was less fat than at other times), eating with either of my parents remained fraught with anxiety. Any discussion of anything edible, never mind the act of actually eating, in the presence of any member of my family still hurls me into a gripping panic that I won't get enough.

A few months after the biscuit-stuffing episode, things had not improved. Although I can't recall any more stuffing-in-secret sessions, they must have been going on because I was getting plumper and I certainly wasn't getting away with eating anything 'fattening' in front of my parents.

One night, at supper, Dad decided to employ a new tack as part of the effort to wrestle my increasing size into shape. Very unusually, the whole family, Dad included, were gathered for a family meal. I'd have been about nine, just before it become evident that my parents' marriage had begun to falter beyond repair.

Supper was mince and potatoes accompanied by some overdone cabbage – standard fare at our house in those days. For Mum, who was becoming increasingly depressed, and for whom the importance of dreaming up varied meals with which to delight her family had never been at the forefront of her mind anyway, the fact that there was anything to eat at all was good enough. I can be more generous now than I felt then about Mum's lack of energy, because now that I'm a mother I've become familiar with the tedium of providing an unrelenting supply of meals for small people who invariably take them for granted. I understand now how unhappy and inadequate she felt.

Once the dishes were on the table, my father stood up, cleared his throat, and said, 'Now, Arabella won't be having any potatoes because she's fat.'

What?! I thought, shocked and surprised. They wanted me to be thinner – they'd made that abundantly clear. But this was obviously a new tactic, a new means of 'encouraging' me to lose weight: public humiliation. It'd always been a great favourite of Dad's: we siblings were always set against each other, being told the other was better at whatever it might be you were trying your hand at, and we were always being compared unfavourably to either each other or other people's much more brilliant children. The idea being, I guess, that we would feel spurred to do better by the idea of being less good than the person we were being contrasted against. My parents were staggeringly competitive – with each other, certainly, but also, bewilderingly, with their children. Dad was always trying to beat us at tennis, bridge, swimming, speaking foreign languages. But then Dad was competitive with the world; it was what made him such a good golfer, tennis player, and skier. It was also the characteristic that ensured he was professionally so successful.

Humiliation had played a big part in Dad's upbringing or rather, as it would have been referred to then, being 'taken down a peg or two'. According to Dad's sister, Lesley, he'd plumped out around adolescence (something he never told us), and this had brought out the worst in their mother, Nancy. Lesley told a story that exemplified this horribly. Dad was 14 when his mother, taking in the sight of his rear, exclaimed, 'Look at you, with a great, big, fat bottom, just like a woman's!' Their mother was a snippy, fierce woman and as such, later, not an ideal grandmother. Nasty teasing from his mother must have contributed to Dad's adult horror of fatness. I'm told Nancy was the life and soul of the party when she was a young woman but she'd been widowed very young, leaving her with little money and two young children, and life was hard for her thereafter which, perhaps, accounts for her unforgiving nature.

Public humiliation, or rather the fear of it, was also probably what drove Dad through an ordinary Fife high school to become head boy and then on to get a scholarship to Edinburgh University. (The Second World War meant he was delayed going to university and, as a result, he went to Oxford instead – unheard of, then, for a Scottish boy.)

Notwithstanding the evidence of my father's success, public humiliation usually brings out the worst in people, and in my case that night, specifically, it instantly made me confused, angry, and, above all, defiant. My unvoiced reaction was, and still is when denied something on the grounds of my perceived ineligibility, 'If you think I'm bad now, just wait: I can be *so* much more bad than this . . .'

So, the potatoes, very much thought of as 'fattening food' in those days, loomed threateningly on the table and Dad was compelled to stop me having any. My eldest brother, Andrew, who was by that stage carrying the chubbiness of an adolescent boy emerging into puberty, sweetly piped up, 'Erm, I'm a bit, erm, you know, and *I've* got potatoes.' I was touched, and I agreed with him. I couldn't for the life of me see why there should be one rule for him and another for me.

But Dad had that query covered and quickly replied, 'That's different: you're a boy.'

What's being a boy got to with anything? I raged silently. Dad hadn't otherwise favoured my brothers over me. He hadn't spent more time with them than he had with me. He didn't do 'boys' activities' with them. In fact, we spent hardly any time with him; he was always at work. I couldn't fathom his ploy; how could being a boy have anything to do with what food you were given? I later understood that it was, in fact, a central part of Dad's beliefs and, to a great extent, Mum's, too. Girls need to be thin and pretty, boys need to be bright – it doesn't matter so much what they look like. Brains for boys do what looks do for women. They both took it as read that an intelligent man has every expectation of being regarded as sexy while the same is rarely true for a woman. However, the unusual element in my particular situation was that *both* my parents were very intelligent and accomplished – that was one of the few things they had in common. They must have known, deep down, that the message being trotted out at supper was deeply unsound and profoundly flawed; but then again, clever or not, they simply did not want and could not tolerate a fat daughter.

Predictably, Andrew's brave intervention didn't help, and I didn't get any potatoes. I spent the rest of the meal seething at the injustice of it all. I hadn't even had a moment in which to work out whether or not I wanted the potatoes; being told I *couldn't* have them, though, instantly transformed them into forbidden fruit and therefore highly desirable.

Occasions such as this and the many others in which various foods were publicly declared off limits to me meant that I ended up unable to assess whether or not I actively wanted the thing. I couldn't consider the food items on their own merit and in my own time. I couldn't think about them neutrally. Eventually and over time I developed a sort of mania: I *had* to have whatever it was because I wasn't allowed to.

This wasn't the first or the last time my parents brought my size and, as they saw it, my need to lose weight to the family's attention; but it sticks in my mind as emblematic of all that was wrong with me. I was wrong for being fatter than anyone else in the family. My parents believed they were helping me by pointing out to me that I ought not to waltz through life thinking it was OK to be me. They thought they were warning me of the pitfalls. As I was, I wasn't good enough. I must learn denial in order to reach a better me and one more pleasing to my parents. The only trouble was that that's quite a tall, if not unreachable, order for a child.

It's hard enough trying to diet as an adult, so tenuous is one's grip in any given moment on how badly one wants to be thin over how badly one wants to eat. And, at the tender age of nine, I wasn't yet up to the levels of self-loathing I'd go on to achieve later in life – the requisite, self-perpetuating levels of self-hatred required to not eat all the time.

This supper was also the first time I remember thinking that life overall wasn't fair. How could it be that I got fatter and my siblings didn't? How was it that they had got automatic membership to the Thin Person's Club, the club that was evidently going to exclude me for life, while I'd got automatic membership to the Whatever You Eat Will Make You Fat Club?

But I learnt to crave food in unnecessary amounts *after* I'd been stopped from having ordinary amounts when eating with the family – not before. I was just destined to be plumper than my siblings. I wasn't doing it on purpose to annoy them. There are scientific experiments where large groups of rats and mice are given exactly the same amounts of food and identical exercise regimes. It turns out that some lose weight, some stay the same, and some gain weight. Well, I'm the fat rat. I'm the rat who eats a Ryvita and puts on a pound. My brothers and sister were the rats who could eat apple pie until the cows came home and never gain an ounce. There's got to be room for all the rats in a family, though, however fat they may be.

I do know Mum and Dad loved me, very much – but not enough to impart the most important message: We'll love you whatever, unconditionally. Their love was more from the 'We love you, but don't be fat, OK?' school of thought.

I can see how they must have felt. I can imagine the difficulty of watching your child increase in size and feeling that something must be done. By monitoring me as they did, they made it clear that it was their pain they didn't want to deal with, the pain of having a daughter who didn't conform, who wasn't gorgeous, who wasn't a winner. But they were not experiencing the very real pain, as it must be, for parents of a genuinely obese child locked into an over-eating downward spiral.

The irony of my parents' apparent willingness to take the bull of my increasing size by the horns was that they weren't dealing with the thing that really needed tackling: their rapidly deteriorating relationship. It was the elephant in the room by comparison with the 'problem' of my weight. But perhaps their marriage – the thing they should have been wrestling into shape instead of me – was too difficult, too terrifying, too impossible, too terminal. Meanwhile, they did have this one issue bringing them together, something providing unity between them: the pressing and, for them, much simpler need to prevent their first-born daughter from getting any fatter.

Too much

Everything changed when I was about ten years old. I can't remember my exact age but I do recall vividly the period, because it was around then that Dad didn't seem to live with us any more. I say 'seem' because, although he'd left London, having gone off to his latest posting as the flamboyantly entitled Deputy Political Resident in Bahrain in the Persian Gulf, no announcement had been made that my parents had actually split up. You'd think you'd remember the day your father moved out – but so much had changed in such a very short space of time. My brothers had gone off to boarding school (and, as it turned out, we never really lived together again); we'd moved to a new house in a completely new area; and I'd changed schools, again. So Dad going to work 3,000 miles away became part of the whole upheaval. And anyway, officially, they *hadn't* split up: the only reason Mum wasn't going out to Bahrain with him as expected, or so we were told, was that she now had a job teaching. Instead, it was presented to us that we would all go out there at holiday times as a family. (This was the late Sixties, when it was still fairly unusual for married women with children, even highly educated ones, to work, so although I appreciate now, from a distance, that Mum was doing something brave and important in terms of realising her own potential for fulfilment, at the time it came across not as a feminist rite of passage but more as an exit from the unsatisfying half-life of being a diplomat's appendage.)

So Mum, my little sister Christina, and I were now at home, in the long-sought-after recently purchased house to which they were both very attached, alone. It soon became obvious that Mum was quite depressed – although the reasons why were much more obscure. (Mum later said she had loved teaching and she was a very popular teacher of English to A level students. However, I don't think she ever felt it was enough of an achievement. Being a teacher wasn't 'good enough'.) I couldn't or didn't ask her what was wrong at the time, as I'd become increasingly frightened of her – not physically, but I could sense her rage all the time. She started shouting a lot, and flying off the handle at the slightest thing. It was around this time that I also began to notice a paucity of food, and correspondingly developed a growing anxiety about how and if I'd get fed. There had been plentiful supplies in the cupboards and fridge when we all lived together, albeit generally off limits to me, but now that the family had fractured, often there just wasn't any food in the house. That can't be an entirely accurate recollection, or else we'd have starved to death, but that's what it felt like. So the association between boys and their

24

entitlement to food was reinforced. No men around seemed to mean that no food was needed.

To make matters worse, my little sister was a waif, a flaxen-haired slip of a five-year-old who clearly wouldn't require as much daily sustenance as the chunky ten-year-old I now was. My very physique – in all its solid difference from that of my little (in every sense) sister – must have felt to my mother like a rebuke, a constant demand to be fed. It is also true that I soon started asking why we hadn't moved to Bahrain with Dad. The constant questioning made Mum furious, but her evasive answers just didn't add up, so I kept on asking.

I have a vivid memory of what little food there was being either covered in mould or festering with maggots. Once I opened the fridge to discover that it was completely empty apart from a lone packet of bacon that was quietly throbbing, so heaving with maggots that it moved as if to an unheard beat. I screamed and Mum appeared and took one look at the offending item before telling me crossly not to be so 'bloody bourgeois'. I had no idea, at that young age, what 'bourgeois' meant, but later realised it was Mum's catch-all way of dismissing anything that was regular, tidy, or conventional. I soon discovered that the whole project of feeding children regularly was also 'bourgeois'. The consistent provision of planned meals was the preoccupation of those too dreary and mundane to do anything more interesting, the kind of people 'who buy fish fingers', my sister and I were told.

That whole unhappy time is encapsulated for me in a scene that took place in the kitchen. Mum was there, in front of an electric, freestanding cooker that, entirely typically of our house, never fitted properly into its designated hole. A gap had been created out of an old fireplace from which the mantelpiece and grate had been removed. The central-heating boiler lived on the left-hand side of the space. In an effort to hide the boiler it had been boxed in, but not very well (again typically and as a result of an attempt to economise), leaving a narrow slot into which the cooker slid. A small, dark, redundant sliver of space remained between the boxed-in boiler and the cooker. It was too small to be useful and just lurked there as a perfect receptacle for all the bits of old food that fell off the cooker during cooking and never got cleaned up.

It was a graveyard for food debris: inches of spaghetti, Bolognese sauce, carrots, stewed prunes, portions of old toast, carbonised bits of lost bacon, an old floret of broccoli, and many other less recognisable scraps of stray food that had escaped from the pans. (These delicacies would all, obviously, have been prepared when the boys were home for breaks from school, not for Christina and me.) And grease, layers of ancient grease, covered the debris and the black-and-white lino tiles beneath. Portions of anything that had ever been cooked on that cooker lay festering in the miniature slipway. Thinking about it now, I suppose you might just have been able to get a brush in there, or maybe a vacuum-cleaner nozzle, but you'd have had to go in sideways, jamming your shoulder right up against the boxed-in boiler on one side and the cooker on the other, all the while trying to avoid the grease that also filmed the cooker's front. It would certainly have been a bit of a struggle and, most of all, you'd have had to care enough to make the effort in the first place.

And Mum didn't care. She never cared about cleaning up. That was bourgeois, too. Later in life, I actually grew to admire Mum's ability not to care about stuff like that. And I only care now because I'd rather have a clean floor than read Proust. If I could choose to care more about reading Important Books than cleanliness, I certainly would. I don't actively want to be the kind of person who puts time and effort into searching the house for dirty cups to make up a full load for the dishwasher. I'd love to be someone whose mind is so packed with great thoughts that they forget to hang out the washing. But when I was a kid I didn't admire Mum's defiant refusal to be house-proud. On the contrary, to an angry, hungry, confused ten-year-old, the filthy cooker 'corridor' summed up everything that was wrong with her. How sharper than a serpent's tooth it is to have a thankless child.

Ignoring the greasy, food-strewn runway, which made me feel sick every time I caught sight of it, I approached my mother. I remember feeling slightly scared, but hunger was driving me on, blinding me to any oncoming danger. 'What's for supper, Mum?' I asked cheerily, hoping the question wouldn't enrage her. After all, we had to have supper, surely?

Mum looked down at me, raised her eyebrows, and drawled theatrically, 'How the fuck should I know?'

My reaction, surprisingly, wasn't fury or indignation or even panic. It was more steely. I remember gathering myself, thinking, OK, right, I know where I am now. In that moment, Mum's response crystallised all the suspicions I'd been harbouring since Dad had gone. I was on my own, and there was no one to help. Specifically, I wasn't to count on being fed. There were meals, of course, but crucially I couldn't assume they'd be either regular or edible.

I now know that, however much she'd thought she wanted it, Mum wasn't coping with her newly single state. She wasn't coping with the house. She wasn't coping with the absence of a sparring partner. She wasn't coping with life. She hadn't ever really wanted to be married – but then, it turned out, she hadn't really wanted to be separated. She had wanted babies but she hadn't really wanted kids. How much worse must her miserable confusion have been made by having small, dependent people making demands for sustenance that she could not meet. Mum simply did not feel she was equipped to cope with it all.

Of course, I must surely have been fed, at least now and again, before and after that episode in front of the cooker. After all, I was alive, wasn't I? And not just alive but noticeably chunky, if the photos are anything to go by. No, I shouldn't have said chunky. Chunky implies greedy, fat, unattractive. Shall we settle, then, on a less loaded description – say, 'not slim'? Unlike my sister, who had those funny little skinny legs kids draw – the ones like two completely unconnected pipe cleaners that stick out of the bottom of a skirt as if they aren't attached to anything at the top.

Later that year, the physical difference between the two of us was publicly paraded – to my utter humiliation – on our first visit to see Dad. Mum, in what must have been an unconscious act of complete madness, used a pattern by

28

Mary Quant (*the* designer of the day) to crochet two identical minidresses in glittery gold silk lamé for my sister and me. By 1968, girls and women of all ages wore miniskirts anywhere and everywhere. It had become a democratic fashion item crossing chasms of class and age. However, it did not cross the chasm of fat. Girls like me, who had more generously fleshed-out legs, tended not to wear miniskirts. After all, there's nowhere to hide in a miniskirt.

Despite her total lack of interest in other domestic arts, Mum was an extremely gifted seamstress and the dresses were absolutely beautiful – simple shifts, sleeveless, with a round neck and falling in a narrow A-line down to a scalloped hem. The perfect shape for a girl with no hips, no bottom, and stick legs. Like Twiggy. And my sister. But not me. Christina looked adorable in hers. She had white-blonde hair cut in a gamine style. On her, it was a suitably fashionable dress that wasn't too grown-up but just grown-up enough to look sweet. In the same dress I, on the other hand, looked like a loaf of bread wrapped in gold cellophane. The dress fitted snugly all the way down. From neck to hem every inch of my body came into uncomfortably close contact with the dress. It was designed to hang off the shoulders and swing gently over a sylph-like form beneath. I looked as if I'd been shrink-wrapped into it. I wanted to die.

I remember Mum laughing as she stood back to survey us both in our new dresses. She wasn't laughing at *me*, but at the stark contrast between how the two of us looked. All the same, she wasn't about to let me change. I pleaded with her not to make me wear the dress. She'd 'sweated blood and tears crocheting that wretched thing', and I was going to wear it whether I liked it or not. And, of course, I didn't like it. How could I? I knew I was larger than most other girls, certainly than my sister. She looked exactly like the picture on the dress pattern; I looked – well, the opposite. What could possibly be more humiliating?

But Mum was immovable, and my sister and I set off wearing the identical dresses – perfect outfits, in theory at least, for a hot, balmy Bahrain evening. We were the new family joining the island's small ex-pat community, and this party was to be our first meeting with the many kids and teenagers from the other families, all of whom had been on the island for a while. And I was making my first entrance dressed as a lump of dough wrapped in gold cheese-wire. Great. My sister was completely, unthinkingly comfortable in hers. Why wouldn't she be? Meanwhile, knowing what I looked like and how my unprepossessing appearance was thrown into hideous relief by how she looked, I began to panic. I could feel the tops of my thighs sweating and rubbing together as we walked. (I once complained to Dad about the horrid, sore red patches that occurred as a result of this. His response was that I should 'push myself away from the table more often'. At the time, I took this literally and could not work out how this 'exercise' would deal with the fat on my legs.) It couldn't have been worse, as far as I was concerned. I was going to a party filled with trendy young people, none of whom, I just knew, would be fat, but all of whom would notice how fat I was – especially thanks to That Dress.

Needless to say the party itself is now a blur, since the all-consuming fear of what I looked like blocked out all possible enjoyment and participation. I do remember, though, that I was right about one thing: I was the only fat kid there. By the way, I'm not suggesting that there were no other overweight kids around in the Sixties but it was definitely more unusual than it is now. Kids now, as we're constantly being told, are bigger than they used to be. (Childhood obesity rates were 5 per cent in the Sixties and Seventies and are now at 17 per cent.) I wasn't obese – well, not obese in the way we now think of it, i.e. as meaning very fat. (In fact, the World Health Organisation's definition of obese is 'abnormal or excessive accumulation that may impair health'.) However, I had more wobbly bits than most of the kids I knew and certainly thought of myself as fat.

It's not that I think Mum made the dresses with the express intention of humiliating me, but I *am* inclined to think that putting me in exactly the same style as my much thinner little sister was some sort of subconscious punishment for being larger – larger in every way, noisier, angrier, hungrier. I certainly felt as though my outward appearance embodied what Mum felt about me – that there was just *too much*.

Daddy's girl

Following Dad's departure, and after a few very unhappy months dominated, as I recall, by awful daily rows with Mum, it was decided that I should join Dad in Bahrain. I don't know who made the decision. I don't think Mum and Dad talked it through – how could they have done, with no phone contact possible? The story goes that Mum came up with the idea because I missed Dad so much. On paper this made sense: I was still a year away from secondary school and not very settled or happy at my primary school. However, it remains in my mind as an extraordinary decision for a mother to make. The very vivid picture I still have is that it came about following yet another violent yelling match with Mum, which culminated in her shouting, 'I can't bear the sight of you any more – you'll have to go and live with your father!'

How accurate a report that is of what actually happened, I can't tell. It is true that we rowed all the time and were both miserable and confused. Me because I didn't understand why Dad had gone away and we hadn't gone with him, and Mum, as far as I understand, because separating from Dad had not turned out to be the instant solution to her misery that she'd expected it to be. It is also a matter of fact that I did go and live with Dad in Bahrain while my siblings and mother stayed behind in England. I can remember, despite the rows, being shocked that she was 'getting rid of me' so easily. I knew I was a thorn in her side, but I didn't know what it was I was doing that pricked her. I only knew that she found me unbearable and didn't want me around.

As it transpired, the few months I spent living with Dad were one of the happiest, if not *the* happiest, times of my childhood. Bahrain is a small island in the Persian Gulf, on the east coast of Saudi Arabia. At that time Western diplomacy was finding its feet in the Middle East. Presumably, with a mixture of sensitivity to local customs and a wish to maintain independence, foreigners lived in compounds. These were made up of a group of houses, some offices, and a pool built by their own architects. They were, by design, little bits of Britain, UK oases in an entirely foreign land. Our small compound resembled a housing estate in the Home Counties. Dad's house was a two-storey, archetypal Sixties – lots of glass and wood – functional box. It had three bedrooms and a bathroom upstairs, with a large hall downstairs, a small study, a living room, and a dining room. There were servants' quarters beyond the dining room, accessed by a swing door like those in restaurant kitchens, which were made up of a kitchen and two tiny bedrooms beyond it. Dad employed two servants: Bundoo and

Bourey, Pakistani men he'd inherited from his predecessor. Having servants might sound terribly grand and from another era, and maybe it was, but it didn't feel like that. With diplomats' budget for 'help', that's just the way it was, particularly for a man with no wife in tow. Bundoo and Bourey didn't wear white jackets with polished buttons, or serve gin and tonics clinking with ice on silver salvers. They were part of the household. I'd often sit cross-legged on the kitchen counter watching them making curries or ironing Dad's shirts or mending or darning – Bourey was a great needleman.

I went to school in Bahrain. The only establishment where the British curriculum was taught was 20 minutes' drive from home and run by the RAF. Dad had also employed a nanny, Carole, to keep me company during the day. The weather was fiercely hot and there was no air conditioning at school, so lessons started at 7.30 a.m. and ended at 12.30, after which I'd go home, have lunch with Carole, and then spend the rest of the day at the communal pool or the beach or riding in the desert. There were very few other children on the island. All the other British diplomats' kids were at boarding schools back home. And although there were a few Forces' kids around – hence the need for the school – they lived miles away in the Forces' compound. There was a minimal public-transport system for locals, but it would have been out of the question for a ten-year-old foreign girl to travel on it, alone. Consequently, I spent all my free time with either Carole or Dad, but I don't remember ever being lonely, or, oddly, missing Mum.

During the time I spent with Dad out there he was indulgent, kind, and affectionate. In fact, he was wholly unlike the dad I'd known hitherto, who'd been remote, hardly ever there, and often bad-tempered when he was. I realise now that this softer dad was a result of a unique combination of things that were true for him at the time: he was still hopeful of a reconciliation with Mum, and uncharacteristically grateful both for my company and, I think, for the opportunity to be a full-time parent to me – something which he surely realised was very likely to end shortly. Perhaps the separation, unofficial though it was, made him more acutely aware of the loss of his children, or maybe he felt guilty about my being out there with no contemporaries; I don't know, but the end result was that I spent more time with Dad than I'd ever done before or ever would again.

And I absolutely adored him. During that time Dad was never critical, never competitive, and always had time to talk to me. Looking back, I think I was Dad's companion as much as his daughter. I was certainly aware of his dependence on me, and this sometimes made me uncomfortable, because I started to worry about him and if he was lonely. It's probably not ideal for a ten-year-old to be in a position where she's looking out for her father's emotional welfare, and this too shaped a lot of my future relationships – but at the time I was just so pleased to be with my beloved father all the time.

Dad's job in Bahrain involved having talks, 'representing Britain's interest', with various dignitaries and leaders from Arab states around the Gulf. Sometimes he'd take me with him. On one occasion Dad was due to make an official visit to a very important man in the region: Sheikh Zaid, the ruler of Abu Dhabi and one of the principal architects of the United Arab Emirates. As the visit was scheduled to coincide with my eleventh birthday, Dad took me along. This was the kind of unworried-by-what-others-might-think, relaxed, loving easy-goingness with which I was very unfamiliar, and it was an unexpected joy every time I experienced it. A tiny propeller plane took us from Bahrain south-east to the Buraimi oasis in Oman, where the Sheikh lived in relative modesty.

After Dad and the Sheikh had had their talk (about the Saudi claim to Abu Dhabi's southern and western territory, I learnt much later in life), our host invited us to join him, his sons, and his entourage for supper. Despite huge wealth gained from the discovery of oil, the Sheikh led a simple, traditional Arab desert-dweller's life. Supper was served just as it would have been for hundreds of years. Dad and I were shown to a long kilim stretched out on the roof of the Sheikh's fort, around which blazed flame torches, embedded into sand, providing the only light apart from the hundreds of twinkling stars filling an inky black, cloudless sky. Three huge unidentified limbless torsos stuffed with rice sat on massive plates equally spaced along the carpet. Between each 'roast' lay plates piled high with delicious-looking rice made with sultanas and pine nuts (I've had that before, I said to myself), plates of okra (I was OK with that, too) and dishes overflowing with what looked like tiny balls of white and black jelly. The Sheikh took his place in the middle and indicated that Dad should sit to his left. Taking my cue from Dad, I settled down cross-legged on the floor next to him, and waited for someone else to start.

Although by now I was familiar with Middle Eastern customs, I had never yet eaten Bedouin-style and didn't want to make a wrong move. A china plate (surely not traditional) sat in front of each place, but there was no cutlery. I wasn't quite sure what to eat or, without cutlery, how to go about it. As Dad was deep in conversation with the Sheikh on his right, I decided to watch what others were doing. Casually tossing his headdress behind him, presumably so that it wouldn't trail in his food, the young man opposite me rolled up his right sleeve and thrust his hand into the hole his side of the beast's torso. He grabbed a handful of rice and then proceeded to scrap the ribcage of the animal from the inside, eventually emerging with a fistful of meat and rice which he plopped on to his plate before helping himself, with the same hand, to the okra and some of the jellied things.

So that's how it's done, I thought, and followed suit. I thrust my hand into the beast and successfully landed some food on my plate. It was delicious: the meat was tender and moist and the rice perfectly cooked. (I later discovered it was camel and that the jellied balls, which I didn't sample, were cooked camels' eyes.) I was hungry and ate some of the okra and flavoured rice happily, too. It was then, for the first time, that I looked up and around at the other guests. The entire company was staring at me. Every single male face was staring at me in astonishment. (In keeping with tradition there were no women present, since the women ate separately from the men – my presence being a gracious concession to Dad.) I couldn't fathom what I'd done to warrant their reaction. Soon, noticing that I seemed to have drawn everyone's attention, Dad looked round at me. Seeing my dirtied hand, he smiled and whispered into my ear, 'You're eating with your left hand; that's the hand they wipe their bottoms with. Most of them will never have seen a girl eat before, and they probably think you haven't got very nice manners.' I made a 'sorry' face to the assembled men, which mercifully was met with some kind smiles and a few laughs. Even then Dad wasn't cross with me.

In fact, this period of living alone with Dad is the *only* time in my life I can remember him not nagging me about my eating habits and my size. It's occurred to me, since becoming an adult, that this might have been because he was low and lonely at the time, and was therefore less inclined to criticise me for something that, after all, didn't matter that much – certainly not as much as a disintegrating marriage. Maybe depending on me and enjoying my company meant that he was less inclined to be constantly noticing what was wrong with me.

Dad and I returned to London together in the summer of 1969 for a family holiday. I also had to start secondary school later that September. Thereafter I'd see him in bursts when he was home on leave, for visits, outings, slightly grim meals in cheap cafés – the typical things estranged dads do with their kids. But in our case it was even more fractured because Dad, as it turned out, wasn't going to live in Britain again until 1974. Estranged dads are bad enough, but long-distance ones, especially in an era of poor or non-existent phone lines and no email, are much worse. From then on I had what you might describe as an on-off relationship with Dad where, it transpired, there was little room for bad times. Seeing Dad very rarely, I soon learnt that best behaviour was expected at all times. There was no tolerance for Bad Fat Me – only Good Thin Me was welcome.

Happiness is a warm scone

During all these early years of upheaval, disapproval, and the growing sensation that I wasn't 'good' enough, there was always Granny She-She, my mother's stepmother. Despite living in Scotland, miles away from London where we now lived, she had a hugely reassuring effect on me.

Every single time I bite into a slice of bread spread with raspberry jam I'm hurtled back into the freezing, stone-floored larder in Granny's house in Melrose. I'm standing close by her as she puts the last touches on the scores of jars she's just filled with her home-made jam. She covers each differently shaped jar, accumulated over the years, with carefully cut circles of greaseproof paper secured in place with a rubber band, followed by circles of remnants of faded material. Each one is then tied tight with old bits of ribbon she's saved. On the top goes the handwritten label: 'raspberry jam', and the year. The jam's still warm and glass around the tiny bit of space between the top of the liquid and the lid steams up. The jam's been made in a 'jam pan' using raspberries Granny picked on her daily walks in the countryside around her house, Eildon Bank. 'There we go, all done,' Granny says, stepping back from the cold stone draining-board that fills the back larder, now covered with jam jars of all shapes and sizes. She puts her arm around me, gives me a loving squeeze, and I draw in that familiar smell of Granny – slightly musty Chanel No. 5, combined with many-times-washed lambswool. Adored and adoring Granny She-She, the first relative to show me unconditional love.

My mother's mother, Eilidh, died when my mother was only 18. The story my mother told was that her mother 'let herself die' once she and my grandfather had retired from the boys' school they ran, apparently saying she had 'nothing to live for without her boys'. At this distance it's hard to know how accurate an account that is. But whatever the circumstances of her mother's death, it's fair to say that my mother, an only child, had always felt unloved and untreasured by her parents.

Mum was brought up in the school – St Mary's, a boys' prep school of about 60 pupils – in Melrose, a pretty Borders town around 35 miles south of Edinburgh. The school had been established by her mother's father in an attractive, large house with generous grounds.

By the time Mum was born in 1926, the running of the school had been handed over to her parents, and she was born in the house. It was a boarding school, and most of the boys saw their parents infrequently, since they lived either in colonial outposts or on remote farms too far away for even weekly visits. Mum's parents took the view that the boys' needs, particularly emotional ones, took precedence over those of their only child, the thinking apparently being that her parents were on hand whereas these boys had 'no mummies'.

Shortly after her mother's death, my mother went to university while her father went travelling to recover from his loss. When he returned he married a childless local woman, Sheila Fairbairn, who acquired a stepdaughter in my mum, whom she cherished right from the start, calling her 'a gift'. And so it was that when Mum had kids, Sheila became, naturally, our Granny She-She, the abbreviation formed by her niece, who'd been unable to pronounce her proper name. Mum's dad died in 1958, but Mum stayed close to her stepmother for the rest of her life. This was easily done, since Granny was the most generous-spirited, loving person imaginable. She was warm, cuddly, and physically affectionate – something that we, aside from during those few early years spent in Innes's care, were not accustomed to. However, she harboured a dark secret, the evidence of which she kept closely guarded – so closely that I only found out about it after she died.

As a family we usually holidayed in Scotland, incorporating dutiful visits to both our grannies. First to Granny Nancy's, Dad's mother in Dunfermline (where we stayed as short a time as possible since she was so difficult and unfriendly), and then on, much more willingly, to Granny She-She's. Later on, from when I was around nine years old and with different school holidays from my brothers, Mum would send me up to Granny's alone.

It is those treasured times I recall best. My mother would put me on a coach at Victoria Station, nervously asking a random old lady if she'd keep an eye on me. An interminable 11 hours later Granny would pick me up in Galashiels, about 4 miles from Melrose, which was the closest the bus stopped to Granny's small town. Coaches were very slow in those days and didn't have toilets on board. Given the cost of coach travel compared to trains, it stood to reason that virtually all the passengers were OAPs, meaning the driver was required to stop every ten minutes for what was graphically announced over the tannoy as a 'toilet visit'. Only the excitement of seeing Granny made the journey tolerable – that, and the knowledge that the kindly old lady into whose care I'd been entrusted would, upon seeing the meagre supplies Mum had given me, take pity on me and share her sandwiches with me or, better still, cake. Those old ladies always had cake – perhaps not the best cake, but cake is cake, especially to a child for whom cake has recently become off limits. Even half a slice of stale Battenburg was always gratefully received.

Mum would grudgingly concede that I probably had to have 'something to eat' during the long journey. She would equip me with a rancid piece of fruit in a wrinkled old plastic bag, still slightly moist inside from God-knows-what, an ancient, smelly Thermos flask filled with watery juice ('not too strong because squash is full of sugar and that's the last thing you need') and, if I was lucky, a piece of sweaty Cheddar wrapped in re-used clingfilm.

But it was all worth it because everything was lovely at Granny's. There she'd be, waiting for me at the bus terminal, with a slightly anxious, searching look on her face until we caught sight of each other, when I'd hare off the bus and throw myself into her arms and she'd squeeze me tightly. Granny felt like soft wool. She always wore the same thing – a 'good tweed skirt, made to last' and a twinset made of lambswool (or cashmere if she'd found a decent second in the local tweed merchants' sale). Granny was healthy and strong from lots of hearty walks, but, like her sweaters, everything about her was soft and giving.

We'd go back to Granny's house on the local bus and as soon as we walked through the front door I could smell the boiled mince and overcooked potatoes. Ever thoughtful, Granny would have prepared the meal before setting off to collect me. Boiled mince and overdone potatoes aren't most people's idea of a lovely supper, but to me this was a feast: hot food in plentiful quantities prepared by someone who loved me and wanted to feed me. Granny's food tasted like what it was – unconditional love. It had all the necessary ingredients: care, forethought, and kindness.

Looking back, what I appreciate now is that Granny loved me enough to think, *in advance*, about what I might need following a whole day's travelling on a coach which reeked of old people's wee. Granny didn't want me not to eat; she expected me to want to eat. Me eating didn't make her cross. She thought I was *entitled* to be hungry. I loved her mince and potatoes. I loved anything Granny made, and some of her cooking was absolutely heavenly.

Nothing in the world comes close to her drop scones, still warm from the griddle, smothered in her raspberry jam, sweet and packed with fruit. And she always made cucumber sandwiches for tea. This was proper tea – cucumber sandwiches, followed by something sweet, usually the drop scones and jam. A proper tea to tide you over until supper. Thinly sliced cucumber sprinkled with a little salt on buttered bread. A snack so simple yet so tasty. When I slice a cucumber now and get a whiff of that fresh, wet smell, Granny's teas by a roaring fire in her living room (even in summer – this was Scotland) immediately spring to mind.

Every morning of my stay, before I woke up, Granny would creep down the windy staircase to the cold kitchen. There was no central heating – she wouldn't have dreamt of going to such an indulgent expense. She'd make two soft-boiled eggs with toast soldiers, accompanied by tea for her and, for me, orange juice in a small can that tasted like aeroplane juice but which I loved anyway. She'd set the breakfast on a tray laid with a linen mini-tablecloth and bring it upstairs, where I'd hop into her bed to eat it with her and chat about what we'd do that day. It was the cosiest, safest place I'd ever been. I was with someone who wasn't irritated by everything I did or said, and who fed me unquestioningly. I was never nervous with Granny, never worried that I might make her cross. She used to say she loved hearing me cry out, 'Granny, where are you?' – explaining that, as she'd never been a mother, she'd never expected to be a granny, and when she heard me call she was reminded of how lucky she was.

Granny's dark secret, which I knew absolutely nothing about at the time, and which makes Granny's capacity for unconditional love and consistent nurturing even more remarkable, was that she was an alcoholic. Granny was drinking so much that she had to get her booze delivered from the next town along, once she'd realised that the store in Melrose had noticed she was regularly ordering an unusual amount. As Granny knew only too well, a small town is a hard place to keep a secret and gossip abounds. Tongues would have wagged, and I could just picture Mrs Laidlaw, the grocer's wife, arms crossed over her pinny-covered bosom, hissing into the ear of Mrs Muir, the baker, 'See, Mrs Walker hasn't had visitors for a good long while but that's another bottle of gin goin' up there with her messages and it'll be the third this week!' It was the norm to do your 'messages' (shopping) by visiting each shop, choosing what you wanted, and the goods would be brought up later in a box. That way there was a fair chance everyone would know what you'd ordered. Granny was a proud person and an active member of the church, St Cuthbert's, situated just behind her house. She sang in the choir and did the flowers for all the weddings, funerals, and christenings. I can't imagine she'd have found it possible to talk about her dependency with the minister.

Yet Granny's drinking never affected my visits. She always seemed calm and in control. We had long walks with her beloved Labrador, Pani, and chatted away to each other happily, never short of topics, mainly the important question of what I wanted to be when I grew up (nurse, pop star, bride, then actress). Granny was never, ever cross or short-tempered. Every night, she'd fall asleep in the armchair by the fire while I watched TV – but all grown-ups did that as far as I knew, drunk or otherwise. So, here was an alcoholic, childless woman of strong Presbyterian faith, that most unforgiving of religions, the only notable joy in her life having been her marriage to my grandfather and the acquisition, thereby, of a cherished stepdaughter and four beloved grandchildren. Yet she harboured no rage, no nastiness, no frustration – outwardly anyway, since clearly the drinking was her antidote to whatever turmoil was going on inside.

Mum adored Granny, too; we all did. But when, after returning home from one of my stays with her, I mentioned to Mum what a good cook Granny was, Mum laughed and said, 'Sheila is many lovely things, but she is *not* a good cook.' I know now that what Granny cooked was wartime British meals, the very meals from which Mum's generation was trying to escape, but at the time I was confused and upset. To me Granny was the perfect cook. She was my idea of that, at least: someone who provided regular food without resentment but instead with enormous love and affection. And, above all, she was happy for me to eat it. This was the complete opposite to Mum's increasingly terrifying reaction to my need to eat.

Cooking blind

Without Dad or the boys around, Mum and I very quickly fell into a pattern of constant, extremely loud, bitter rows, punctuated – intermittently – by miserable meals invariably provided with rage and resentment.

But when the boys came home from boarding school for visits, Mum always made an effort. Suddenly, there'd be fresh bread, a variety of salamis, meat, lovely cheeses, salads – you know, proper, nourishing food. And if they happened to be there still on a Sunday, we'd sometimes get roast chicken followed by apple pie. However, lest I give the impression that my brothers never experienced Mum's whimsical approach to food provision, let me recount the following story.

I've already said that Mum wasn't a bad cook; in fact, she was extremely accomplished but only when she chose to be. She was knowledgeable about good-quality ingredients and was capable of producing an impressive variety of complicated dishes. However, in the Sixties the fashion for feeding children the same-quality fare as adults hadn't yet evolved, at least not in Britain, so my awareness of Mum's skills mainly came from being around when she prepared for dinner parties while she and Dad were together, or on the very rare occasions she gave them once they'd split up. Her culinary talents were hardly ever wasted on her kids. Except for one memorable day when the boys were home from school.

It was lunchtime and Mum announced that she'd made some 'delicious lentil soup'. Ah. Now, this would be a good few years before the lentil had managed to shake off its reputation as the unremittingly dull pulse of choice for the kind of hippies who baked bread using their own placenta and wove their own shoes out of bark. Back in 1968, only Claudia Roden and a tiny minority of truly talented cooks well versed in the exotic ways of rendering a lentil palatable could possibly have dreamt of eliciting a positive reaction from four recalcitrant children who were already slightly wary of their mother's idea of 'delicious'.

In one synchronised movement we all slumped our shoulders as Mum plonked down the pale brown, lumpy slop in front of us. (My kids, at 10 and 11, around the age I was then, have taken up this physical means of showing displeasure. 'Not pasta again!' they moan and it makes me want to scream 'Yes, bloody pasta again!' – even though my starting point is not one of frustration, loneliness, and desperation. It can't have been much fun for Mum.)

Of course, us doing this made Mum cross, crosser even than her constant default mood which was ... cross. 'It's delicious, and what's more you'll like it!' she yelled. We all peered nervously down into our bowls. It certainly didn't look delicious. In fact, it gave every sign of being utterly revolting. I was sitting next to my sister and opposite both my brothers at the kitchen table. Mum had gone back to the cooker. We exchanged worried looks. 'What are we going to do?' We couldn't eat it; that much was obvious. Andrew, always the peacemaker and, it has to be said, the one least likely to spark Mum's rage, fell on his sword. He picked up his spoon and tasted the soup. Emboldened, Matthew, Christina, and I gingerly followed suit. As we had suspected, it was absolutely foul.

We dropped our spoons, which clattered noisily back on to the table.

Mum spun round. 'What's the matter? I spent hours making that, and you're bloody well going to eat it.'

We knew better than to put up a fight. One by one we picked up our spoons and tried again, but we couldn't get it down. It didn't just taste horrible in an infantile all-lentils-are-yuck way. It tasted wrong. The soup had a tangy fizz – surely *that* wasn't right?

'Is this what lentils are supposed to taste like?' I hissed at Andrew.

He furrowed his brow and hissed back, 'I don't know. I don't think so, but she's going to go nuts if we don't eat it all.'

He continued, bravely, with tiny spoonfuls, while I resorted to clanking my spoon about in the bowl in the hope that somehow this would reduce the level of the soup and convince Mum I'd eaten some. Mum's rage could flare so suddenly, and you could never be sure what would spark it.

We didn't know how we were going to get out of this.

Then it happened – sudden, blissful, unexpected salvation. Andrew summoned up his courage. 'Mum, I think there's something actually wrong with this—' But before he could finish his sentence, as if by magic, projectile vomit shot out of his mouth and nose, travelling at speed right across the kitchen table. The jet was so strong, it looked as if it had come out of a fireman's hose. No one said a word.

As the last regurgitated lentils dropped off Andrew's chin, Mum marched forward and picked up his spoon to taste the soup. Never one for apologies, she chose her words carefully. 'Yes, very well, the lentils *might* have gone off, but it *was* delicious when I made it.' Thanks to Andrew's super-reactive stomach, unbelievably, we were off the hook.

I've since grown to like lentils (only when they're fresh) but I still can't eat them without instantly recalling the fizz they emanate when they're off. But I'm not sure any child genuinely likes them. I made some delicious (no, really) lentil soup the other day and even persuaded my kids to taste it. My daughter went first, before urging her younger brother to try, too, but 'not to look at it before'. He wrinkled up his nose: 'I'm not being rude, but I think that's more of a grown-up's type of thing.'

I don't think, for one moment, that Mum knew the lentils were off or that she was deliberately trying to poison us. Very irritatingly for her, they'd simply gone off since she'd cooked them, so, operating in the belief that she had something to give us kids, she suddenly found herself a meal 'down', as it were, and I can certainly relate to how bloody maddening that can be. You know you've got to feed your kids, find that the intended meal is sabotaged, and now have to find a substitute. An unfortunate episode such as this might be a small hiccup, hardly worthy of mention, to someone for whom cooking for their kids is no big deal; but if your default position is one of anger, resentment, and frustration at where you find yourself in life, as was Mum's at the time, then it's small wonder she was so pissed off. Those lentils exemplified Mum's hatred of cooking and the insurmountable drudgery that it was for her. They also illustrate that we were not accustomed to food being prepared with love and care. Our food, such as it was, was angry.

Shock in awe

I dare say few children caught in the crossfire of a dissolving marriage remember it in terms of what they ate. But I do. I think, probably, that's because food provision – or lack thereof – in our house was so concretely linked to the overwhelming, harder-to-pin-down feeling that every single thing was now unsure, unreliable, and shaky. That nothing could be relied on. Mum and Dad weren't officially separated: with the family holidays still being spent in Bahrain, they had them to hold up as 'proof' (to themselves as much as the outer world, I suspect) that they were still a functioning couple. However, Mum was melting down, Dad was withdrawing, and meals were hit and miss. Food became the symbol of the multitude of things that were going wrong. For me specifically, of course, food and entitlement to food were 'not allowed' – and they became the embodiment of all that was wrong with my life and me. So, although I realise my siblings felt the break-up deeply from their own perspectives, for me it will for ever be linked to my weight and its management.

There were times when Mum's, erm, breezy attitude to her children's need to eat resulted in downright farce. One of the most memorable happened on one of the last family holidays our parents attempted before finally admitting they'd actually split up.

Dad was home on leave and had borrowed a cottage on Loch Awe in the north-west of Scotland from a fellow Scot at the Foreign Office. Despite it being summer, the weather was grey and damp. All the same, in keeping with my parents' hardy upbringing, we'd go for long daily walks ('Stop moaning, it's good for you'), tramping over hill and dale for what seemed like hours and hours. As a child Mum had been made to sleep with the window open every day of the year and take a morning bath in two inches of cold water. Although Dad hadn't endured the bath regime when growing up, also being Scottish he certainly shared the same Spartan approach to parenting. Mum didn't want to go on these walks but she knew we ought to, while Dad actively enjoyed gruelling exercise. The lone highlight of these enforced treks was the strawberries and raspberries that grew wild away up the hill. We used to gorge ourselves on them – fresh, incredibly sweet, and bursting with flavour. To this day I can't taste a strawberry or raspberry without instantly bringing that holiday back to mind.

Every night, as convention dictated, Mum was called upon to produce a meal for the four of us children. She and Dad ate together later, a 'grown-ups' dinner'. Things being as bad as I later found out they were, I don't know what –

if anything at all – they could have talked about when they were alone. It must have been extraordinarily hard for them both, but particularly Mum, who still didn't know what she wanted from (or without) Dad.

One evening, ordered to help with supper, I joined Mum in the kitchen and watched with mounting nervousness as she wrestled with an unfamiliar and unwieldy can opener, struggling to get some unlabelled tin cans open. After a great deal of characteristic effing and blinding she finally succeeded and began to shake the contents into a pan.

'What is that?' I asked tentatively.

'I don't bloody well know! The labels had come off. The supermarket didn't know, either, so they sold them to me for a penny a tin.' Her response didn't exactly fill me with confidence. Neither did the gloopy, jellied, can-shaped substance that slithered out into the pan. It certainly didn't look very appetising. 'Some sort of meat, by the looks of it,' Mum declared, shaking the second can's contents into the pan.

'But what kind?' I ventured.

'I don't know. Doesn't matter, does it?' she replied briskly, clearly not expecting or wanting a reply. (I dread it when my kids ask me what's for supper only because the reaction is usually a complaint of some sort.)

Once it was heated up, Mum spooned the stuff on to four plates piled high with mashed potato. It didn't look great. We took our plates over to the Formica table without which no Sixties kitchen was complete, sat down, picked up our forks, and hoped for the best. My first mouthful immediately came shooting out of my mouth so fast, Andrew had to duck to avoid being hit by it. It was completely revolting and bore no relation to any animal any of us had ever eaten. Andrew, undeterred by my reaction, put a forkful in his mouth. Out came missile number two. This one landed on the edge of his plate.

'What the devil's going on?!' Mum shouted. To be fair, it must have looked as though we were 'exchanging fire' on purpose.

'This isn't meat. It's weird. It doesn't taste right,' Andrew piped up.

Now, I don't know if it was because Dad was there and, perhaps, Mum was happier, or if she was just in a sunnier mood – or maybe she'd had to put so little effort into making this 'meal' that she was more prepared to be relaxed about the reception with which it was met. Whatever the reason, and very uncharacteristically, she hesitated. Having already admitted she hadn't known what the cans' contents were, she didn't have the full force of righteousness on her side.

At that moment Dad sauntered into the kitchen. 'Finished already, have you?' he drawled in his teasy way, as if we were taking a breather between the endless courses of a gourmet feast.

We all sniggered conspiratorially. Dad had broken the tension, and even Mum cracked a smile.

'Mum bought some cans of meat for a penny each, but we can't eat it,' Matthew blurted out.

Dad wandered over to the bin where the denuded cans lay discarded. He smelt the inside of the can, and recoiled.

We were on the edges of our seats. Dad turned the can upside down and read the information printed in tiny letters on the bottom. 'Mmm, little wonder it's not to your tastes. It's dog food.'

Released by Mum's guilty smile and Dad's knowing look, we all immediately fell back from our plates, flamboyantly mimicking the death throes we'd seen in a million shoot-'em-up movies, our mouths dropping open, limbs flailing everywhere, clutching our stomach, and jerking theatrically. 'Bleurgh! I'm going to be sick!' 'That was in my mouth. I'm going to die!' 'I'm going to puke!' Determined not to be outdone, Andrew 'swooned' to the floor, while Matthew opted for convulsions, grasping his throat and uttering desperate strangled noises, the victim, clearly, of a dastardly poisoning plot.

'Very funny,' Mum said drily, arms crossed, leaning up against the counter. 'You can leave the meat, but you're still eating the mash. I'm not making anything else.'

We couldn't believe it. What kind of mother would expect her own beloved offspring to eat mashed potatoes infected by dog food? We were lost for words. And hungry. We looked down at the plates in disbelief. 'Suit yourselves,' Mum trilled, knowing she'd won. 'Don't know what you're making such a fuss about anyway. It might be dog food, but it's still meat.'

Scots of my parents' generation weren't brought up to *enjoy* food. Why, the very idea goes against everything that is Scottish, Presbyterian, and 'good for you'. Life is not about the pursuit of happiness but the pursuit of goodness, and thinking of others before yourself, always. You have only to have sampled porridge to know that. I'm well aware that porridge has had a renaissance in recent years, but the porridge I grew up with was made with water and salt. Need I say more? Porridge as I knew it is the culinary equivalent of a hair shirt. It wasn't designed to be tasty and enjoyable, but to sustain life, a shoulder to the wheel, no more and no less. Food in general was only there to keep you alive. The notion that it might be fashioned into something tasty and delicious was completely alien, and doing so could surely only lead to gluttony, to *eating for pleasure*. It'd be a helter-skelter slippery slope after that. Who could tell what random wantonness would come next? Sex for pleasure, no doubt!

Both my parents had been brought up to respect parsimony above all else – something that goes hand-in-hand with simple and modest consumption. Predictably, once away from their parental homes and Scotland, both my parents quickly found a taste for the good things in life, specifically alcohol and good food. However, they never acquired the ability to feel entitled to such indulgent luxuries, as they continued to see them – or, moreover, to equip their children with a relaxed sense of entitlement and expectation where food was concerned. It wasn't until I met Jewish families that I understood meals could be delicious, plentiful, and available to all in equal measure – that they needn't be measured out in portions according to who was most in favour, or most deserving by dint of their size. In other words, that a family eating together could be an expression of love.

Funny valentine

It had already dawned on me before becoming a teenager that my burgeoning roundness made me harder to love. There was certainly plenty of evidence that this might be the case, since what I ate was under perpetual scrutiny and my parents got cross if I ate and showed pleasure if I didn't. So naturally it followed that to make them less cross, i.e. to love me more, I ought to eat less – in front of them, at any rate. However, tying up love with eating makes for a tortured and very complicated mish-mash of two very basic human needs that ought, for a child at least, to be completely separate from each other and free of any burden of guilt.

This is easier said than done if you come to parenting carrying a whole gamut of unsorted-out problems, particularly if they happen to fall in the area of self-esteem and you haven't even begun to unravel them. Parenting is, after all, a relentless internal battle between, on the one hand, desperately trying not to project on to your beloved child all the problems you have and, on the other, stopping them from making mistakes you feel sure will plague them for life. And evidently being fat was, for both my parents, akin to being disfigured.

I don't think anybody would suggest that either of my parents, at this stage in their lives anyway, was blessed with the ability to be self-analytical or self-critical, so what they thought tended just to tumble out, irrespective of what effect it might have on me. In fact, I think when things got too much for them they were subconsciously compelled to offload their own feelings of insecurity, vulnerability, and fear on to their children, with the frantic but unspoken message that 'This is too much to bear, I don't want to experience the pain of this feeling, help, yuck, you have it.'

One February, when I'd just turned 12 and wasn't yet in the grips of full-on teenage angst and sulking, I innocently wondered out loud, in Mum's presence, whether I'd get any valentine cards. Looking back, I don't know where I'd have got the idea that it was even a possibility. I was in my second term at an all-girls' school and hadn't yet met any boys, really, except a few of my brothers' school-mates, and I can't seriously have imagined that any of them were going to send me a card. It must have been that I'd been caught up by the whole marketing bonanza. But on the morning of Valentine's Day, to my huge surprise and delight, a card addressed to me arrived in the post. I was fit to burst with excitement. It was a beautiful, cream-coloured card with a big red heart on the front. Inside was blank, save for a question mark and a single cross, a kiss.

I rushed off to show it to Mum, who looked pleasingly surprised and happy, while I immediately started to speculate about who might possibly have sent it. It was my first-ever valentine and I was naturally thrilled by it, but also by what its arrival had ignited. I was now able to dream about someone (albeit unknown) liking me in 'that way' enough to go to the bother of anonymously letting me know. I was filled with the excitement of trying to work out who my admirer might be.

But this was a step too far for Mum. Having to witness me, her young, not conventionally pretty daughter, in a flurry of innocent hope and pride, breathlessly musing out loud about who, from the handful of boys she knew, might really fancy her, was too much for Mum to endure.

'Oh darling, don't. I can't bear it. I sent it,' she suddenly blurted out, looking at me with a pained expression.

'What?' I stuttered.

'I sent it to you. I couldn't bear the idea of you not getting any. I knew you wouldn't, so I sent you one.'

I was crushed. 'But why are you telling me?' (Although I was deflated, I'd instantly worked out that if she hadn't told me then that wouldn't be the case. I would just never know.)

'Because I can't bear listening to you wondering if you've got a secret admirer when you haven't.'

'Oh.'

'Oh darling, don't be upset. That'd be silly. You wouldn't be feeling like this if you hadn't got so excited by it all,' Mum added, not very successfully trying to smooth things over and, as ever, shift the blame and her own discomfort. She'd set out to do a nice thing but – once faced with the real-life consequences of my reaction to her ruse – found *she* couldn't cope with the way that made *her* feel.

It wasn't just Mum, though. Dad too found it difficult to separate his own feelings from my responses, which added to the confused and confusing messages I received about the inverse relationship between my size and my lovability. One evening in particular sticks in my mind. Before Dad left the family home for Bahrain (as it later transpired, never to live with us all again), he, Mum, and I had established a night-time routine that I really enjoyed. At bedtime my parents would come up to my bedroom to chat while I got into my nightdress and then they would kiss me goodnight before leaving the room. But one night, out of the blue, Dad left the room, and stood in the hall outside with his back turned.

I asked Mum what was going on. Looking embarrassed, she mumbled that Daddy wasn't going to be in the room any more until 'after' I'd got changed. I was very perplexed, and asked what I'd done wrong. 'Nothing,' Mum replied, not looking at me. 'Just leave it. I can't explain. You'll understand when you're older. Daddy's just going to wait until you've got your nightie on.' I remember too that, having struggled unsuccessfully to explain the situation, she then shot Dad a cross look over her shoulder. Dad didn't see it, though, and I'm not sure what it was intended to convey other than that she was annoyed at having been left alone to deal with this difficult moment.

So, as far as I could tell, they were both cross about something and I couldn't work out what it was. I was ten at the time and not showing any signs of approaching puberty.

But I was plump. And I was upset that from now on Dad wouldn't be in the room for the chatting I liked so much. So, with plenty of evidence to support my train of thought, I worked out that, since he could be there before I got undressed and again when my nightclothes were on, what must be wrong was the bit in between: me naked. As I wasn't yet experiencing any of the innate wish for privacy that accompanies the onset of puberty, I wasn't at all grateful for Dad's withdrawal. And, as nothing had really been explained except the hope that I'd understand when I was older, it stood to reason that I'd blame myself – or rather, in this case, the way I looked, since that was the only thing that happened in the moments Dad was electing to be absent.

Obviously, I did work out later that Dad had anticipated, wrongly, that I'd start showing signs of becoming a woman soon, and was trying to be sensitive before it all started. But at the time, and for years afterwards, I assumed that the intolerable, unbearable thing, the thing Dad must avoid seeing, was my body – and clearly that was because it was too fat.

I tell this story not in an effort to catalogue my parents' faults but to explain, I suppose, how difficult my weight 'problem' must have been for them. If a few minutes of my hopeful excitement at the thought that someone fancied me, or a fleeting glimpse of my pre-pubescent nakedness, was too great a load for either of them to bear, then no wonder they couldn't cope with the ever-present issue of my size. It was too hot a potato for them to handle.

. . . and under her veiled glance
I felt my bosoms and bottom
swelling up through my head. I
was so conscious of their size and
presence, they could have toppled
me off my legs.

Good Behaviour by Molly Keane

My other family

I was very lucky because early on in my life I met a couple whose influence became a major contributory factor in taking the edge off my combative relationship with Mum and my general sense of not being 'good enough'.

In the spring of 1970, through one of my new pals at secondary school, Cathy, I met Toby Reisz, a boy she'd known at primary school. Free of any of the adolescent awkwardness caused by mutual attraction, for which we were anyway a bit young, we hit it off immediately. Toby was funny, energetic, and quick-witted. His parents were divorced and, when we met, his mother was in the process of moving to America so, unusually, Toby and his two brothers moved into their father and stepmother's house. Their dad, Karel, had been born into a Jewish family in Czechoslovakia but was sent to England as a boy to escape the Holocaust, in which his parents died. Now completely anglicised, he was a film director, and Toby's step-mother, Betsy, was an American actress who'd worked in

Hollywood before being blacklisted in the McCarthy years and moving to Europe, where she met Karel.

Betsy and Karel, who had no children together, presided over an astonishingly relaxed, bohemian, comfortably off household into which I was warmly welcomed from the very first time Toby brought me home. I had never met anybody like them before in my life. They were, of course, glamorous by dint of their jobs, but in a completely unshowy, unintimidating way. When I followed Toby into their enormous kitchen-living room to be introduced to his father and stepmother that first time, any nerves I had were dispelled instantly; you simply couldn't be nervous around them. Nothing about them called for anxiety. What Karel and Betsy did for a living was incidental to the big-hearted, expansive, friendly atmosphere that prevailed in their home.

The thing that struck me straightaway was how pleasantly tolerant they were of the boys and their friends. There was never any shouting or yelling, or even objection to the hours and hours of lolling around in Toby's room we indulged in, not a few years later more often than not smoking dope. In fact, there was never any evidence of what a nuisance we might have been. We didn't seem to irritate them by just being ourselves. I was not used to this. Even more amazingly to me, I was always invited to stay for supper. And to my further astonishment we all ate together – Toby, his brothers, and I were positively welcome at the table. Adult delight in the presence of young people was completely unfamiliar to me. I was used to my company (particularly when eating) being a visible irritation. I'd become used to being regarded as annoying. Yet here was a family who were willingly including me, who actually wanted me there.

And the food was always fantastic, plentiful, and tasty. Dishes from Karel's childhood were often produced, I think, to remind him of his lost Jewish heritage – classics such as red cabbage stewed with vinegar and raisins, white cabbage stewed with caraway seeds, apple strudel, and proper, good-quality frankfurters. And there'd always be old-fashioned American staples, from Betsy's 'portfolio', such as meat loaf made with ketchup (it's *really* good baked) and pot roast. And we were *encouraged* to eat. I wasn't pitted against the other children, no comments were made about whether I ought to be eating certain things, and no one rolled their eyes if I had seconds. Other, more interesting things were the topics of discussion. Ample amounts of good food were simply presented as part of a loving, inclusive atmosphere. Rather than what I had become accustomed to – which was the provision of food for children being a necessary evil, a nuisance, and something to be dispatched as quickly and minimally as possible – in the Reisz household it was the very reason we, the kids, were brought together with the adults. They actually wanted to have their meals with us.

Here, suppers weren't made up of a ragbag assortment of foodstuffs at various stages of putrefaction; there were no decomposing dishes in the last stages of rancidness; there were no dirt-encrusted vegetables (Mum regarded washing food before cooking as 'bourgeois' and you learnt to be on guard for a mouthful of rock or a lump of earth when you bit into a potato at our house). There were no disgusting things, many moons past their best, laid out with the guilt-inducing charge that they 'must be finished off'. Despite being of the same generation as my parents, Karel and Betsy shared none of their abstinence-equals-good mindset. Karel and Betsy believed in hard work and realising one's potential, but they didn't believe these goals were achieved through suffering, denial, and social embarrassment.

Meals at the Reiszs' were freshly prepared, varied, and always heavenly. And I found all this incredibly liberating. To put things into perspective I ought to mention that they had a cook, the wonderful Carmelita, originally from the Philippines, so little wonder, I guess, the whole feeding-kids assault course was so hugely different there to how it was at my house. Carmelita provided regular and reliably available food to which I was always welcome – chicken with noodles and vegetables and special fried rice were particular favourites for all of us. This effortless approach to feeding kids and eating as a family was a complete novelty to me and felt like untold luxury. This overwhelming sensation of warm, open inclusion, coupled with my friendship with Toby (and eventually his brothers as well), resulted in my spending more and more time at the house. As the years went by I became friends with Karel and Betsy independently of Toby – something that further validated my sense of self-worth. In many ways they were my surrogate parents, my 'good' parents, as it were.

With hindsight, however, I am very aware that it was much easier for them to be all that they were to me than it was for my mum. They had a happy marriage and interesting and successful careers; they were very much where and who they wanted to be in life. That was the exact opposite of where Mum was in hers, despite the fact that she was otherwise in every way their intellectual and social equal. Also, including me in their world wasn't a daily task. I'm conscious of how easy it was for me to idealise them, and, although they were my sanctuary, I know now that a comparison between them and Mum is not comparing like with like.

And as my relationship with the Reiszs grew certain elements were introduced, particularly later, when I became an actress, and then it wasn't entirely stress-free. Once I'd started acting, Betsy – misguidedly rather than meanly – introduced a new element: monitoring how I looked. Starting out as a novice, I took part in all and any crappy, unpaid fringe production I was offered. Betsy would very loyally come to see me, without fail and often alone, in these inevitably dismal shows. Before too long she began to offer me advice. Being very unconfident about what I was doing, I eagerly welcomed her tips about how to commit to a piece even if I thought it was dreadful. (Apparently one could tell what I thought of the play from the audience – not good, seeing as I thought most of them were shit.)

But then came the hints about losing weight if I were 'serious about making it'. Although I was crushed that my precious, 'perfect' surrogate mother had stooped, as I saw it, to my parents' level, Betsy's 'help' ought to be seen in context. Unlike my parents, who were motivated by *their* feelings about having a fat daughter, Betsy was motivated by the belief that all actresses *had* to be thin to succeed. And she was right. All my generation of actresses were young, pretty, and thin. There were no fat ones, very few black or Asian ones, certainly no disabled ones, and hardly any working-class ones, either. It appeared that all actresses of my age were drawn from one teeny-weeny section of society populated exclusively by white, thin, and unusually pretty posh girls.

It was embarrassing and agonising when Betsy suggested I should start seeing Karel as a 'director first and friend second' and dress accordingly when visiting their house. At the time no one, including me, would have been able to predict that, in fact, being comfortable the way I was would be my only hope of success. But Betsy wanted Karel to give me a job. She wanted to help me out. As she saw it he was a film director and I was an actress. He had the power to bestow on me work that could, might make a big difference to my burgeoning career. (Karel did eventually give me a tiny part in one of his movies, *The French Lieutenant's Woman*, but I don't think he could ever have seen me in anything beyond that.)

And the important difference when Betsy nagged me about my weight was that she never once made me feel that I'd be less well loved or less welcome if I didn't conform – whereas that is what I *always* felt when under attack from my parents. In this, my other family, I got to be part of the gang for exactly who I was, not a girl who needed to be thin and pretty, which, for a good sense of self, proved invaluable and exactly how it should have been.

A waist of time

After Bahrain Dad was posted to New York to make up part of the British delegation to the Security Council at the United Nations. Following this move my parents dropped all pretence of still being together. Mum and I still weren't getting on but there were fewer hysterical, fever-pitch rows, perhaps because things between her and Dad were clearer now and we all knew they'd formally split up. More immediately important to me was that, to my surprise and huge relief, I was popular with my peers at my secondary school (if not my teachers) and very happy.

Two girls in particular, Sophie and Sue, became my closest mates early on. Sue was the first person I'd ever met who was thin and pretty but still insecure. I'd never thought such a thing was even possible before I met her. Hitherto I'd understood, and been led to believe, that being thin and pretty was the answer to everything. How could someone so pretty, slim, and beautifully dressed (Sue always had the most fashionable clothes) be unsure of themselves? Luckily for me, from the very first day of school, we recognised in each other identical, hidden feelings of not being 'quite right', and it bonded us from the outset. Hard as it may be to believe now, divorce was fairly uncommon in those days, so the fact that Sue, Sophie, and I were the only 3 girls out of 90 fellow pupils whose parents were divorced meant we were a breed apart, or at least felt like one.

In addition to that unique status, Sophie offered a different kind of bond from the one Sue and I shared. Just like me, Sophie was plump. She and I were the two roundest girls in a year populated exclusively, it seemed, by pencil-thin girls with gangly long legs and shiny, silky hair. We quickly realised not only that we both struggled with our weight but that our parents had very similar views on their daughters' sizes and what we ought to be doing about it. This combination ensured we became staunch allies in the 'war on weight', and from our early teens we embarked together on mad, pointless, sometimes near-starvation diets.

Up until then we'd been the victims of action taken by our parents in an effort to reduce our weight – action that we resented and rebelled against. But now we embraced the brilliant discovery that we could deny ourselves food. We saw controlling our own food intake as giving us positive command of our own destiny. We were no longer being starved by our parents in pursuit of thinner, more socially acceptable daughters; instead, we starved ourselves in pursuit of being more fashionable and popular with boys. The fashion icons of the day were young, slim women such as Twiggy and Sandy Shaw, we were reading *Jackie* magazine, and the revealing miniskirt was all the rage. The irony was that Sophie and I weren't heavily overweight at all. However, if you didn't look like an approximation of the stars of the day, you felt yourself to be huge. There were absolutely no normal-sized girls out there, no big role models, no visible women who were in any way 'bigger' than the girls on the catwalk or the hot-pant-wearing dancers in Pan's People or even those appearing in the audience on the dance floor in *Top of the Pops*. There was one shop that catered specifically, and not fashionably, for larger girls, and it was called Evans Outsize. With that name, it might as well have been called Fat Pigs.

So with absolutely no idea what we were doing, no diet book and no information about nutrition or age-appropriate calorific intake, we hastily calculated we could live on about 800 calories a day. We'd worked out that this figure could easily be achieved, since neither of us got fed very much at home (though Sophie's mum was less resentful about meals than mine), and the rest of the time we were our own masters when it came to controlling what went into our mouths.

We started this new regime by stopping school dinners, even though I secretly quite liked them. Even then I knew I was supposed to be snobby about mass-produced, over-cooked food. I knew I was supposed to find it revolting, but I didn't. These meals were hot and plentiful, available without comment, and I could get pudding – and that still adds up to my idea of a great meal.

This was the early Seventies, before television and magazines were inundated with experts talking, writing, and making programmes about good food being an essential 'lifestyle' necessity; there were fewer opportunities and less pressure to be snooty about food. Still, it wasn't that I liked school dinners because I thought they were quality food. Even then I could distinguish between old cabbage boiled for six hours in a vat of old water and flavoured with a truckload of salt, and lightly steamed fresh, young cabbage rendered super-tasty with butter and interesting herbs. But eating for me was, and probably always will be, more about availability than quality. Just as it was with Granny She-She's meals – how could they ever be revolting, even if overcooked, unseasoned (salt and pepper was about as exotic Granny's cooking ever got) and not particularly varied? They were hot, there, and served with love. Granted, our school dinner ladies probably didn't love me, but they didn't seem to care (or even notice) if I had pudding – oh, those wonderful, sticky, doughy, jammy, completely-free-of-any-dietary-merit puddings unique to schools!

The only gauntlet I had to run was the derision of my friends. Out of our trio – Sophie, Sue, and me – Sue was the only one who could not eat school dinners. She had been brought up by a mother who cared about food, cooked well, and – a complete novelty to both Sophie and me – thought her kids were entitled to eat as well as she did. And Sue was never fat. Before the dieting began, when at school mealtimes Sophie and I piled our plates high with absolutely everything on offer, irrespective of what it looked like, Sue used to struggle with the idea that we'd contemplate eating something that wasn't nice just because it was there. What I wouldn't give for that mindset! That's the mindset of someone who believes they're entitled to eat good food and, what's more, expects it. That's not the mindset Sophie and I had.

Now, though, mindful of our 800-calories-a-day marker, and with all the demonic zeal unique to converts embarking on a new mission, Sophie and I agreed to bring in food to share at lunchtime. Sophie had found a little booklet that had come free with her mother's copy of *Cosmopolitan*. It was a small yellow thing, similar in size to Chairman Mao's 'Little Red Book' (which was also popular in the early Seventies – possibly more intellectually en-riching, but of less use to two dieting schoolgirls). It was called *Your Handy Handbag Calorie Counter*, and you were advised to 'keep it with you at all times' so that you could 'quickly check the calories' of every single thing you might consume. What fun! Dieting women did things like that in the Seventies. It spoke to their commitment to keep trim. Women everywhere would produce pocket-sized reckoners and sit, with a plate of food in front of them, working out how many calories it all added up to. And they were not ashamed to be seeing doing this. Society then and now applauds a woman on a diet.

To set the scene, here are some of my diary entries of the time:

9.1.71 I must start slimming on Monday.

20.1.71 Must slim.

26.1.71 I must slim.

16.2.71 I really haven't got any willpower, I must get slim.

At school and for a long, long time afterwards, I didn't think about whether dieting was a good idea, either personally or in a wider sense. I just wanted to be thinner.

Our lunches every day were a hard-boiled egg, one each, a small pot of warm cottage cheese (it had been in our lockers all morning) to share, and some cucumber. We could have as much cucumber as we liked, since Sophie couldn't find a calorific tabulation for it in the booklet, so we decided it must be calorie-free. In fact, we soon decided that anything completely taste-free and very watery had zero calories. Take celery, for example: somebody told us at the time that it was actually calorie negative – so indigestible was it, the theory went, that it took your body more calories to burn it off than the amount of calories it contained. We were thrilled with this news and quickly added celery, which neither of us liked, to our daily repast.

We didn't think it mattered that we didn't like most of what we were eating. That wasn't the point. Anyway, we were sure that you weren't supposed to like the food you ate when dieting – in fact, the less you enjoyed the tiny amounts of food you allowed yourself to eat, the better you did, because then you might eat even less of it because it wasn't nice. See? We were forging ahead to the Holy Grail: being thin. We had the hallowed ground of being slimmer in our sights. We were being Good. We were resisting the temptation to indulge and therefore 'without sin'. We certainly were not in the business of simply eating less of the food we actually liked – that would have been akin to rewarding ourselves, and that would have been like healthy eating! That would have been the action of someone with a balanced attitude to food. That, in fact, would have been the approach of someone who was very unlikely to go on a diet in the first place.

So, celery, boiled eggs, and cottage cheese, day in, day out. Oh yes, plus – how could I forget? – some Ryvita: about two, maybe three, pieces each. They actually tasted OK – which we feared meant we were bound to have to 'pay' for it somehow – and, according to the booklet, they were 32 calories a slice. We'd started out with a stiff, dark brown strip of Swedish crispbread called something like Kunderklap or Smogersbrat, Shitshton. Whatever its name, it looked like how it tasted: a flattened-out, hard-baked turd, petrified by time. It promised everything it delivered: a month's-worth of chewing to dispatch it, and a desert-dry mouth upon completion. Not even we were prepared to surrender to this much misery in pursuit of its low calorific count. On the plus side, you could have loads of them, since they were lower in calories than Ryvita. However, committed as we were, after some sterling efforts we eventually succumbed to Ryvita's superior taste, not to mention its capacity to be digested.

Every day Sophie and I would hole ourselves up in a corner of the cloakrooms, laying out our meagre feast.

'So,' Sophie would say, her mouth filled with egg, '80 cals for the egg, erm, what do you reckon, 'bout 125 for the cottage cheese, that's . . . er . . .'

'205,' I'd chip in. I was completely useless at maths, but better than Sophie.

'I knew that, so 205, plus two Ryvitas at 32 cals each, 64 plus 205, er . . . Don't say anything, 269. That's not bad, 269 for lunch. We've got over 500 cals left for supper.'

'Yeah, but you've got to include something for the cucumber and celery. They can't really be completely calorie-free.'

'S'pose so. A tiny bit. OK, let's call it 300 for lunch.'

'Yeah, definitely,' I'd inevitably concur. 300 calories sounded pretty good.

On the way home, after school, lolling along casually, walking in that painfully slow, sloping way unique to teenagers, Sophie and I would usually buy a Curly Wurly from the sweet shop behind school. Everyone got sweets to eat while walking home. Somehow the Curly Wurly never got included in our calorie round-up. We didn't really count it. It didn't appear in the booklet and why would it? Dieters don't eat Curly Wurlies. Chocolate doesn't even exist for dieters, so why would its calorific content appear in the dieter's bible? Also, so went the reckoning at the time, as we were eating it while walking, we were probably burning off all the calories as we ate. Occasionally, as we strolled along, Camilla, one of a pair of impossibly pretty and universally popular twins, would annoyingly pipe up, 'Aren't you two supposed to be on a diet?' Sophie and I would exchange guilty, conspiratorial glances and either snarl at her ('MYOB') or look virtuous and reply (lying), 'We're using up our supper allowance on them.'

As you might expect, when it came to sports we were both uncomfortable and reluctant. Usually we managed to get away with doing nothing, since the teachers clearly had no interest in making girls participate who they knew were going to do badly on purpose. However, one day a particularly courageous PE teacher, Miss Little, spotted Sophie and me huddled in the corner of the sports field and selected us to go first on the hurdles. We thought she was joking. PE teachers never picked us to do anything. But this one was going to make us take part. She was going to make us take those hurdles if it killed her.

Apart from the occasional rounders match, neither of us had ever done any kind of sport. We hadn't the faintest idea how to clear a hurdle. We literally had no clue how one got over them.

We approached the line and just stood there, shoulders slumped, as if facing a brick wall. As Miss Little barked, 'Ready, steady . . .' Sophie and I doubled up with hysterics, shoulders shaking with laughter. 'Go!' Exchanging one last grin, off we ran, heading straight for the hurdles. With no idea of what to do, we attempted the first as best we could. One little fat leg stretched out in front of us, attempting an approximation of a right angle to the setting-off leg, body bent over, desperately attempting to simulate the sort of lunge that might just clear the hurdle. We weren't trying to please Miss Little, we weren't trying to excel in hurdles. We were genuinely trying to clear them: they looked as if they might really hurt if you went into one broadside. And they did. In unison, Sophie and I brought down every single hurdle we charged. Twelve hurdles smacked straight into our thighs, each one as forcefully as the last. We collapsed in howls of pain, clutching our reddened thighs, and scowling as meaningfully as we could at our PE teacher.

This is how our lives went for years and years. Every single lunchtime we diligently counted calories. We'd lose some weight, and then there'd be holidays and we'd put it on again, or one of us – well, both of us – would eat something prohibited when out of the sight of the other, so up and down we'd go. It hardly mattered, though. We were best pals, united by divorced, dysfunctional parents, and being overweight. We were never teased about it – our gang wasn't really like that – but all the same we never got used to being fat. And we certainly never got comfortable with it.

Kurt Waldheim finds out I'm fat

The futile (as it eventually turned out) quest of constant dieting was a predictable stage given how much attention had been paid to my weight in the years leading up to my teenage years. Along with every other teenager who has ever lurked around moodily, feeling hard done by and misunderstood, I had all the ultimately meaningless (yet at the time massively important) insecurities and worries that beset all kids at that age, plus the added dilemma of knowing I was fatter than most of my contemporaries – or maybe I should say rounder. Though most pre-pubescent girls carry puppy fat, as it's affectionately known, I not only had more – dog fat, it should have been called – but it didn't leave as I grew (I've still got it!). Little did I realise then, however, when embracing the notion of limiting my intake of food in order to reduce my size, that I was actually embarking on nearly 30 years of yo-yo dieting, fruitlessly investing fresh hope and wild dreams (not to mention money) in every new, miracle, guaranteed-to-work-this-time diet launched on to the market.

When I started dieting in earnest I was, of course, also entering puberty, a journey which for any teenager, irrespective of gender or sexuality, is linked to the usually torturous process of considering how, if and when one becomes sexually active – which, in turn, is inextricably coupled with becoming super self-conscious about your looks. For me this whole physical and emotional maelstrom was further complicated by the fact that Dad was becoming sexually active as a single man. Thankfully, I don't know exactly how active he was, but it was pretty clear that he was 'on the market'. The transition of little girl to pubescent daughter is a tricky time for most dads and daughters, but I think it's fair to say that it's even more thorny for the daughter if circumstances force her to become aware of just how sexy her dad is at the same time.

In New York, the epicentre of all that is happening, exciting, and ever changing, and keeping company with intelligent, sophisticated movers and shakers engaged in the highest levels of international diplomacy, my father was in his absolute element. And why wouldn't he be? He had recovered from the break-up of his marriage and had thrown himself headlong into single life, with great results. Within a few months of arriving he was being pursued by slews of glamorous women all keen to bag themselves a 'Roger Moore'. (I remember several of them cosying up to me in a way that, even at 13 years old, I could tell was phoney, and clearly done only in an attempt to endear themselves to Dad.) And he now drove a sports car – well, sort of: a Ford

Capri. British diplomats were required to drive UK-made cars in order to 'fly the flag'. The Capri was the closest thing available within his budget that was sporty. So, aside from having what I regarded even then as a slightly naff car, Dad was every bit the smooth, handsome, and eligible bachelor. One can well imagine how, having been lonely in Bahrain and rejected (as he saw it) by Mum, he might savour his new suave self. He was reaping what he'd sowed. The 'fat' boy from Dunfermline was living the high life.

As a direct consequence (at least, that's how it felt at the time) of all these exciting opportunities, Dad was also much less of the indulgent father he'd been when we lived together alone in Bahrain. I suppose he no longer regarded me, at 13, as a dependent child in need of her father's affection and protection. However, I did, naturally, still need his approval – in fact, even more so than before, since I was seeing much less of him and felt increasingly peripheral to his new, action-packed life. This anxiety was reinforced by Dad making no secret of preferring me thinner. He didn't seem to question the preference or his motives. He simply informed me that he was prouder of me and loved me more if, when I went over to see him, there was less of me.

Although both my parents had gone on about my eating habits and the need to be thin, it seemed to start mattering more to Dad at the stage when I was a developing teenager. Perhaps I mean more *specifically* to Dad. Mum was just in a state of rage with me all the time about everything – my poor academic performance at school, my stupidity compared to her friends' daughters, anything and everything that I liked and she didn't approve of. So Mum nagging me about being overweight, painful though it was, felt like another thing in the catalogue of stuff she didn't like about me. Whereas Dad, whom I now only saw sporadically, focused particularly on my size when we met. I suspect he wanted an attractive, slim 'little lady' kind of a daughter to show off at parties more than the daughter I actually was – a plump, insecure, stroppy one. For stroppy was how my personality was shaping up. In lieu of being a swot, I'd quickly established myself as the class clown, armed with ever-ready wise-ass quips for teachers who dared to control or confront me. From the very first day of secondary school – a place where, for the first time in my life, I knew I'd be staying after years of moving from one school to another – I had instantly worked out that if I couldn't conform and blend in as one of the normal-sized, pretty girls from an ordinary family of non-divorced parents and 2.4 children, then I'd have to go that extra mile to stand out and make the most of being 'different'.

Thanks to the up-and-down and largely unsuccessful dieting, during the years that Dad was in New York my weight fluctuated dramatically. Every time I visited him I'd be a different size. On one occasion, when I was 14, I flew over for an early summer visit. I was fatter than I'd been the last time we'd seen each other and, as I walked through the arrivals' gate, I could see the disappointment on his face. He didn't say anything but I knew. Of course I knew. Dad had been pretty clear about it being 'better' if I was thin. As we climbed into his car – the low-slung, racing-green Ford Capri – I could sense his disapproval. It felt as if my fatness was filling up the whole space, squishing into every inch of the car's neat little cockpit.

During the visit, we drove up to Massachusetts one boiling-hot weekend to attend a lunch party given by the Urquharts. Brian Urquhart, then the Under Secretary General of the UN, was a very old friend of Dad's. Sydney Urquhart, Brian's American wife, was a tall and elegantly beautiful woman whose home and marriage appeared to be all that was refined, smart, and enviable. From my perspective, the Urquharts had the perfect life. Their parties were always populated by the great and the good and, notwithstanding the trek up from the city, this lunch – a barbecue around the lake by their idyllic Shaker farmhouse – was no exception. One of the guests whose presence I soon had particular reason to recall was Kurt Waldheim, the then UN Secretary-General.

For some reason, I was the only young person at the party. The Urquharts had three children, one of whom was around my age, but none of them was present, which was maybe why the other peoples' kids weren't there. This shouldn't necessarily have been a problem. I had become accustomed to being Dad's companion at adult events. I'd got used to doing that in Bahrain. In fact, I'd loved it. On this occasion, however, I was clearly supplementary to requirements: Dad neither showed me off nor needed me as a prop. He'd probably have preferred to go alone. And being the lone teenager meant there was no young crowd into which I could blend. To make matters worse, since it was a lakeside party, everybody, including me, was wearing a swimsuit.

Not yet fully neurotic to the extent that I'd sooner have worn a burka than a bikini – that fever-pitch level of neurosis took a few years to finesse – on this day I was, quite innocently, wearing a bikini. This is not, I now know, the ideal outfit in which to eat if you're uncomfortable with your body, and especially not if you have a few 'spare tyres'. There's too much exposure, literally, too much opportunity to spot the evidence of what you've eaten already in your life. But I wasn't thinking like that yet. I wasn't yet scrutinising every single thing I wore for how much of me it revealed or accentuated, flatteringly or otherwise. I was just wearing a bikini, the sort of swimsuit anyone my age would be wearing. I hadn't thought about the dangers that lay therein.

On a long table covered by a pristine white linen tablecloth sat bowl after bowl of delicious salads, rice dishes, potato dishes, sauces, cold cuts, cheeses, bread and crackers – everything you could possibly need to complement barbecued food. The table occupied the entire length of the beautifully manicured lawn around which the guests milled, drinking and eating. No one was paying particular attention to me. I was hungry, and quickly decided that this was an ideal opportunity to get something to eat, unnoticed.

I took a plate from the pile and walked along the buffet, selecting various bits of the mouth-watering spread. Having helped myself to a bit of everything that took my fancy, I picked up a serving spoon and leaned across the table to scoop up some rice salad which lay towards the back of the buffet. Suddenly, I heard that withering drawl I knew so well boom out across the lawn (you wouldn't think it was possible to drawl and boom simultaneously, but it is): 'Rice *and* potatoes, darling? Is that a good idea?'

As one, the assembled guests turned to see where Dad had directed this comment. Me. In that instant I suddenly saw what they must be seeing: an overweight teenager in a bikini (for God's sake!), a roll of fat cascading over the top of her bikini bottoms like uncooked bread dough piling over the sides of a baking tin, clutching a heaving plate already piled high in one hand and with a spoon laden with rice salad in the other. I must have looked like the cherubic Cupid posed to strike a new lover, but in extra large, and sporting a plate and spoon rather than a bow and arrow. I was sure they all shared one single thought: Might it not be best if she wasn't eating at all?

I immediately froze in that position – I didn't dare to put the plate or spoon down for fear of drawing further attention to myself. I was poleaxed with shame and embarrassment. Like a kid caught with a hand in the cookie jar, I thought that by not moving a muscle I might somehow not actually be noticed after all. My plan didn't work. Eventually, I lowered the laden spoon slowly back into the bowl of rice salad. As I did so the overloaded plate wobbled in the air as if it had just found a voice and was screaming, 'There's too much food on me!' I stood stock still, bent inelegantly over the table like a podgy garden statue, my still-outstretched arm clutching the quivering plate almost audibly groaning with food. I felt as if my exposed flesh had run riot and was taking over the entire garden. Tears of shame pricked my eyes. Then, suddenly, I exploded, and yelled 'Fuck off!' as loudly as I could, inadvertently including

Kurt Waldheim in the full blast of my attack. Unfortunately for him, he was standing right in the line of fire between Dad and me. I hurled the plate back on to the table and marched off into the house.

Sydney followed a few minutes later and found me convulsed in tears. 'I told your father he shouldn't have done that. He's sorry.' I was very grateful for her support and, although I had guessed Dad would be a bit sorry, I also knew he'd meant what he'd said. After all, he'd been well schooled in the art of teaching someone a lesson through the medium of public humiliation.

Despite my indignant rage and mortification I, of course, believed deep down that he was right. I shouldn't have been (nor should be now) eating rice *and* potatoes. Good Me, the Real Me, wouldn't even *want* two lots of carbohydrates, never mind actually consume them. Bad Me knows they taste great and wants to eat both of them. Good Me might, at worst, sample them, but would be able to leave it at that. Bad Me wants them and eats them – and, what's more, in sizeable quantities. This is typical of one of the many internal arguments that anyone who puts on weight easily will have with themselves at least once a day. We watch ourselves every minute of every hour even when we're not officially on a diet. It's like installing CCTV in your head which you can't switch off – ever.

Dad loved me, of course, but with conditions, with an ever-present 'room for improvement' caveat. He was, I now think, embarrassed, and probably ashamed, too, that his daughter was not only fat but wearing a swimsuit that didn't attempt to hide the fact and, on top of all that, brazenly eating in it. I don't think Dad was able to summon up the internal confidence required not to feel that it was, in fact, he who was being judged for having a daughter like that.

By commenting publicly on the inadvisability of having both 'rice *and* potatoes', Dad was immediately deflecting attention away from himself and his potential complicity in my 'bad' eating habits. Figuratively speaking, he'd jumped up, pointed at me, and shouted to the assembled crowd, 'Look, I know she's overweight! Don't judge me! It's not as though I want her to be like that!' I know Dad wasn't deliberately trying to expose me to ridicule. But I suspect his main aim was to rid *himself* of the discomfort he felt watching me eat 'too much'. Just as importantly, he'd have felt compelled to head off any possible criticism from his fellow guests of his failure to police my eating rigorously. Dad had worked very hard to get into the 'winners' enclosure' and he had every right to be there. However, I don't know that he ever truly felt he belonged. Even today it would take a huge leap for a Swotty Horace (as he was known at school) hailing from a very unremarkable town in Fife to feel he was truly at home in high society. My view now is that he always felt extra pressure, albeit from within, to have all the conventional trappings of success – and a chunky, rude daughter certainly does not rank amongst these.

Of course, I didn't understand any of that at the time. All I felt back then was that in order to be really loved by Dad I had to be thin and pretty. Later that day, on the way back into the city, I managed to mumble some sort of complaint about what he'd done. He replied, as if in mitigation,

'What can I do? I like having pretty girls around me.' I remember thinking that that didn't sound right. I wanted to reply, 'Aren't I just supposed to be your daughter, not some pretty girl?' But I didn't. Tellingly, however, Dad didn't tell me off for having sworn loudly at him in front of his friends and colleagues, so, I guess, he must have known he'd brought it on – a bit, anyway.

It's hard enough on kids when parents break up, but there's an added and uniquely difficult aspect to it all when the relationship with the estranged parent is long distance. The child never gets the time or space just to 'be' with that parent. I felt as though I now had to earn his love, and to do that I had to be on best behaviour at all times. Time together was too limited, too precious, to waste on being anything other than charming, compliant, and attractive. It was made clear that there was no room for the sulky, flare-wearing, rebellious, fat teenager.

All you can eat at the boy buffet

In the summer of 1973, six months before I turned 16 – and contrary to everything I'd learnt (or, one might say, been taught) up to that point to expect – boys starting paying me attention. Not all boys, not every boy I met, but more than one – a few, enough for me not to think it was by accident.

At first I couldn't compute it at all. I was still plump. I wasn't huge, but I was definitely chunkier than all my pals, yet here were boys clearly fancying me. How could that be? Boys don't fancy fat girls. Fat girls don't get cool boyfriends. *Nobody* likes fat girls. I knew this was true because of how my parents behaved and because that's what we got from TV shows, magazines, newspapers, movies – the message was everywhere. All the pretty girls are thin and they're the ones who get the good-looking, cool boyfriends. Girls who eat aren't lovable. I knew this to be true for I was not.

The fat girl is there, sure, but she's the funny one, the best mate of the pretty girl, the tomboy, the one the guys talk to as though she's not a girl, as though she's one of them. And I was all of those things. By this time, I had become the clown, in and out of class. I could always be relied upon to be the naughtiest in any group and to do the most daring things. I was – had to be – the funniest, the one who jollied things along. This was how I expected to get attention. But I was still overweight, so how could it be that I qualified for the much coveted, incessantly talked about, all-important attention from boys? I didn't get it. And I wasn't the only one to whom it was a surprise.

Among the boys who fancied me was one who was properly cool and tasty. Nick was a trendy, handsome boy of 17, two years older than me. He had long hair, a moped, and corduroy trousers, and he rarely spoke. He was everything every girl looked for in a boy. Quite a few of our gang liked him but I was the one he asked out. One of my school pals, Camilla, unanimously agreed to be ravishing, mused out loud, 'I can't believe Nick fancies you if he knows I'm available.' I agreed with her.

So I went out with Nick and discovered that he liked me in spite of my being fat. Well, I assumed it was in spite of it, because he never said anything about it. He can't have not noticed or not thought it. I never got used to it not being an issue for someone else, someone who was keen on me. How could it not be? Since I knew I wasn't lovable except when I was thinner, I couldn't get used to the idea of being lovable as I was.

And after I broke up with Nick there were other boys, lots of boys, who fancied me. Incredibly (literally, to me), I turned out to be quite popular. But I never stopped waiting for the axe to fall. I kept waiting for each boyfriend to mention the fat. They didn't. But I worried constantly about how I was getting away with it. On a practical level, one way I swerved from detection was to make sure I never stood up in front of any boyfriend when in the nude because, as I saw it, once he'd caught sight of me like that he'd instantly realise why I couldn't be loved. My fat stomach and droopy breasts would naturally be the corporeal evidence that I was unlovable.

So what actually happened, aside from my managing to conduct all the unclothed elements of my relationships from a horizontal position? Did I embrace this bewildering new stage of admiration and draw from it the lesson that I actually was likeable and sexually appealing, even if plump? Did my self-esteem rise accordingly, blossoming with every new boy who showed interest in me?

Of course not. Programmed as I was to think that I wasn't entitled to any of this, that I didn't deserve the stuff other people got, that I hadn't earned it – and just as with food – I gorged myself. I ate, as it were, as many boys as I could. All in an effort, I guess, to see if their interest was real, if this could really be happening to me. Since I was confident that nothing I offered was reason enough to pick me out of a crowd, I kept sampling every new boy who liked me – partly in disbelief that no one was trying to stop me loading up my plate from the boy buffet ('Rice *and* potatoes, darling?'), and partly because I was sure that the feast would be whisked away at any moment and without warning.

How I felt when responding to boys is summed up in something that happened when I was about eight years old. Someone had given me a chocolate bar. 'I like chocolate,'

I said once I'd eaten it. Quick as a flash Mum replied, 'But chocolate doesn't like you.'

Just as when I stuffed myself with biscuits, bread, or any other food I'd been told I wasn't supposed to eat, I never took time to evaluate each individual boy on his own merits. I simply responded instantly to the fact that the boy was there, offering himself up to me. I never once stopped to think about whether I wanted him. I would never have expected him to wait while I considered my interest in him. I seized him, as it were, because he fancied me. As I believed my appeal wasn't based on anything solid (in fact, it was clearly in spite of quite how 'solid' I believed myself to be), naturally I thought that if asked to wait he'd immediately lose interest. I believed myself to be easily dispensable. Exactly as with food, my fevered response was always, 'This is a one-off, it won't be here tomorrow, you can't rely on this, grab all you can now!' In essence, the easy availability of boys or food is a once-in-a-lifetime opportunity that you must snatch in that moment or lose for ever.

Also, and anyway, I never rid myself of the suspicion that I'd *made* the boys like me, that they couldn't just have liked me of their own free will. I was always talking, joking about, drawing attention to myself. I put a huge effort into being likeable, and therefore when someone did like me I secretly feared it was only because I'd made them do so. Of course, I then feared that if I relaxed and was just 'me' from the start, no one would notice me at all – and they certainly wouldn't get the idea of fancying me because I was intrinsically unfanciable. So it was my job to make people like me.

And oh, the satisfaction when I met someone who was openly disapproving of my size and eating habits yet at the same time prepared to suffer the ignominy of going out with me. I say 'satisfaction' and mean it, but in a religious, self-sacrificial way like wearing a hair shirt or having a cross to bear – he's going out with me even though he, as he ought to, thinks I need to be thinner. That way I could outsource my own feelings about my size. So, when and if a certain boyfriend was particularly mean, I didn't have to 'own' any of my own discomfort about my size. I could make it entirely about what a wanker he was. I *gave* him/them (they're were actually three, would you believe, consecutive disapproving boyfriends – a hat-trick) licence to behave that way. I allowed them to demean me, criticise my eating, shape, etc., because it meant I was back where I belonged, in the familiar role or rather family role of being told I was fat. Wankers as they arguably were, they couldn't have behaved like that unless I'd let them, given them permission to do so. I had the real power veto (I didn't have to go out with them, after all) and handed it to them so that I'd be free of the responsibility of caring or not about my weight. They, just like my parents, had taken on responsibility for it by being unpleasant to me about it. Result. I found people who would reflect back to me that I was as undeserving as I believed myself to be. I wasn't going to make the mistake of going out with someone who actually liked me and didn't think there was anything wrong with my size! Hah!

This mania falls under the umbrella of insatiable hunger, for food and attention – they both come from the same place. I ate (and still eat) when I'm not hungry, and I slept with boys I didn't fancy to keep them fancying me. It wasn't and isn't about sating a genuine, identifiable hunger. It's about trying to fill an unfillable space – the void that's created when you don't believe you're entitled to anything in the first place. It's about not being equipped to take your time and select something with confidence. And this is an easily reached view for girls, with or without food issues, now just as much as when I was young. If the universal view is that popularity with boys is king, then how do girls develop the intuition, never mind the right, to pick and choose what's best for them?

My fairy stepmother

On one of the holiday visits to see Dad in New York, when I was 15, at his suggestion I brought my friend Sue along for company. Dad was going to be tied up at work in the UN most of the time I was there, so it was felt that having a pal with me would mean we could travel around together doing various different things in the city during the day. We happily travelled on the subway going to shops, exhibitions, and open-air concerts in the park, enjoying the huge, exciting variety of things New York in the summer has to offer. Most evenings Sue and I would have dinner with Dad or tag along with him to the many parties to which he was invited.

One evening Dad threw a party at his apartment. Some of the guests were non-diplomatic-service friends he'd made since arriving in America and others were colleagues. One woman, Hilary, a junior colleague from the British representation at the UN, was noticeably younger than most of the other guests, who were, in the main, Dad's contemporaries. She was tall, very slim, pretty, and, I remember vividly, noticeably very nervous when introduced to me. And I sensed straight away why.

A little later, I followed Dad into the kitchen as he went to get more ice. 'That woman in the other room, Hilary, she's your girlfriend, isn't she?' I asked nonchalantly, leaning casually against the kitchen counter. I was trying quite hard to make this sound like just another topic of inconsequential conversation. I was very aware that Dad had been seeing other women since splitting up with Mum, but he hadn't yet formally, or at least publicly, started a relationship with anyone significant.

Up until then I had intuited who was after him, using as my never-fail gauge how unusually keen they, grown women, were to talk to me, an (at that stage) deliberately uncharming teenager. But Hilary was different: there was something instantly appealing and unpushy about her. She clearly genuinely wanted me to like her, rather than it being a tactical ploy to get closer to Dad.

'Erm, who? No . . .' Dad replied clunkily, cracking ice trays over the ice bucket. I knew he was lying.

'Yes, she is,' I persevered. I could just tell. His evasiveness only added to my certainty.

'No, she's not . . .' Dad continued, unconvincingly, 'but, anyway, do you like her?'

That was it. I knew it. He'd hardly want to know whether or not I liked her if she wasn't his girlfriend. 'Yeah, she seems nice.' I had taken to her, but suddenly thought I ought to pull back and pretend she was no more than one of Dad's guests. Mum and Dad weren't yet divorced and he clearly wasn't about to go public with this relationship. I didn't want to flush him out into the open with it if he wasn't ready. And I didn't want to get the sharp end of Dad's tongue. If you ever pressed him on something it turned out he didn't want to talk about, be it pocket money, overpriced (as he saw it) birthday presents, or going on holiday alone, he didn't kindly steer the conversation another way, allowing you a way to back out. Like as not, he'd go on the defensive and bat you off with one of his favourite remarks ('Can you really be as stupid as you look?' or 'Do you ever stop to think before you open your mouth?'). Dad could be withering and haughty and you pushed him for information at your peril.

That brief meeting with Hilary took place in the summer of 1973. Dad was posted back to London at the end of the year and I can't say I thought about her again until a few months later, on one of my regular weekend visits to Dad's tiny, slightly dismal rented flat. He was busy on the phone so, bored, I started to poke around his bedroom (undetected, naturally). Deliberately hidden from view was an invitation addressed to 'Michael and Hilary'. So, just as I'd thought, she had been his girlfriend, and still was. Hearing Dad end the call, I quickly put the invitation back where I'd found it, wondering how serious this relationship was. Dad was a secretive man at the best of times, added to which he and Mum were, I later found out, having huge difficulties agreeing on a divorce settlement.

It wasn't until another year had passed that Dad, with a great deal of hesitation and shifty lack of eye contact, announced he was moving into his 'friend Hilary's flat'.

I honestly think Dad thought calling her his 'friend' meant that I wouldn't know they were lovers. Very soon afterwards my sister and I were invited to supper. I don't remember what Hilary cooked for us other than the roast potatoes she made, which were absolutely sensational: perfectly crunchy and oily on the outside and fluffy and moist inside – the best I'd ever tasted in my life. We instantly warmed to her. She was really nice, genuinely kind to us, and could not only cook very well but seemed to do so willingly, happily, and easily. These attributes continued to make up a huge part of how beloved she became to us.

Soon after they'd moved in together, they married. This was a very difficult time for Mum, who still wasn't very fulfilled or at peace with herself. I suspected that she didn't really harbour any serious hopes of a reconciliation with Dad – I'm not even sure she wanted that – but nonetheless she sadly told me that she felt she was being 'left behind'. Painful (and arguably inappropriate) as it was for Mum to offload this on to me, her child, I understood because I felt the same. Dad was marrying a woman 20 years his junior with whom he was going to start married life all over again. Where would we, his first family, fit in?

But, as it turned out, there wasn't a single moment in which those fears were able to take hold since, from the very start of their marriage, Hilary made superhuman efforts to include and welcome her four stepchildren – and, incredibly, Mum – into their new life.

After separating from Mum, Dad had continued to join us for Christmas at the family home. My first fear after Dad and Hilary married was that this would stop and inevitably we wouldn't see him 'for presents' on Christmas Day any more. Even though I was 19 by this time, it still meant a great deal to me to be with Dad on that day. Occasions such as these, like birthdays, become symbolic for kids whose parents separate – you sort of cling on to sentimental markers and over-invest in their meaning. It's yet another indication of how out of kilter your emotions can get, and this is especially true when your parents' break-up is messy, unclear, and drawn out.

Hilary had evidently anticipated the pain of this possible wrench and, despite being pregnant with their first child, invited us all round for Christmas lunch – Mum, too. Mum and Hilary actually had a great deal in common. They were highly intelligent, well-read women with strong personalities, and crucially they hadn't been rivals. For all Mum's ability to be very immature when she wanted to be, she knew that Hilary had nothing to do with her break-up with Dad. Mum quickly grew to appreciate Hilary's many wonderful qualities, in particular the unconditional love she showed her stepchildren, and also how much more emotionally accessible and present Dad became to all of us under her influence – an infinitely better father. It wasn't long before Dad and Mum became friends again, and they both knew they had Hilary to thank for making that, the once impossible, possible. And I think it's fair to say that our stepmother made our dad.

Over the years, Hilary was always an extremely supportive, fair-minded, and kind sort-of-parent. Although she never tried to take a parent's role, telling me what to do or disapproving of decisions I'd made, she supplied many of the most welcome things that parents, particularly mothers, provide – such as hot, plentiful food, a patient, attentive sounding board, and an ever-necessary conduit to our often impenetrable, unreachable dad. And, unlike those of both my parents, Hilary's feelings for me didn't seem to change in accordance with my continuously fluctuating weight.

Hilary was undoubtedly the perfect stepmother as much as she was the perfect wife – too perfect sometimes, in my view. For she could also be very exacting and bark alarming demands for detailed information on your plans for, well, anything from something as huge as your career to what you were thinking of making for a supper with friends. But whilst her line of questioning could be terrifying, she always meant well. Belying her enormous generosity of spirit and kindness to others, though, Hilary was very hard on herself. She demanded of herself perfection and therefore took any criticism as justifiable comment, particularly if Dad was its author. One occasion, for me, exemplifies this perfectly. Hilary not only worked full-time, baked her own bread, took the dog for early morning walks, and bicycled all over town but made an at-least-two-course meal every single night. One evening I visited them both for supper. (The two boys they'd had together by this time were away at school.)

During most of the meal Dad, as was his habit, read the paper, leaving Hilary and me to catch up. Once we'd cleared away the plates (Dad still reading the paper), Hilary produced a delectable-looking pudding, a portion of which she put before Dad.

He peered over the edge of his paper down at the bowl, and then looked up at his wife, his face screwed up in disdain. '*Bought* pudding?'

My stepmother replied, 'Yes, sorry, the thing is, I had done a—'

This was too much and I jumped to her defence. 'Dad, "bought pudding"? Are you bloody well joking? You should count yourself lucky you're getting pudding at all!'

Although I don't think he thought he should have been given 'bought' pudding, Dad did laugh. And Hilary did believe, like many, many women, that to qualify as the 'perfect' woman (to which we're all striving, obviously), she should not only have a high-powered job but also produce a hearty meal for her family every single night – and that includes a home-made pudding. Despite being a whole generation younger, Hilary was beset by the same self-doubts endured by my mother – as she was, she wasn't 'good' enough (and this seems to be a common malaise for women, especially mothers, even today. Not the 'have it all' generation but the 'do it all' generation – that's us).

Yet in many ways, Hilary was cut from the same cloth as Granny She-She: hard on herself but wonderfully generous and kind to others. Completely unlike Dad and Mum, who externalised all their problems and anxieties into criticisms of me and others, my stepmother turned all her self-doubt and worries in on herself – just as Granny had done. While I'm not, by any means, advocating inward thinking or self-punishment in a parent or carer, or anyone for that matter, I am extremely grateful that, whatever ailed Hilary, she didn't feel compelled to visit it on me. For all her relentlessly unforgiving demands on herself, tellingly, Hilary – who was extremely thin (and mystifyingly fearful all her life of becoming fat, even though she'd never been overweight) – was always sympathetic when we talked about my worries about my size and never judged me for my inability to lose weight, despite being able to command such incredible self-control and discipline in herself. She couldn't tell Dad to get lost when he criticised her for buying dessert rather than making it, but she could have a go at him when he voiced the opinion that I shouldn't be eating nuts, potatoes, or pudding at all – which he did, without fail, on every occasion we ate together, and this didn't stop once I'd become an adult or once I was a mother. Every single time we shared food, whether it be a biscuit with tea, nuts accompanying drinks, or a sit-down meal, Dad would draw attention to my 'right to eat'. He just couldn't help himself – 'Darling, did you know,' he'd drawl, 'that nuts are very fattening?'

Eventually, after Dad had died, Hilary did manage, little by little, to share some of her anxieties with me, and before her untimely death of cancer at 63 years old, just over two years after Dad's death, I think we'd become even closer than we were before. I'd like to think that I was, for what turned out to be the tragically short time remaining, as good a friend to her as she was to me for more than 30 years. Although she came into my life too late to temper Dad's constant monitoring of what I ate or to make a difference to how I felt about myself physically, she did affect an immeasurably huge shift in how I dealt with Dad and his endless criticism of my size. Dad and I ended up having a much easier, more loving relationship than we'd have been able to have without Hilary's influence, I'm sure. And for that, amongst so much else, I will be eternally grateful to her. Hilary united a disjointed family.

When I first went into the movies Lionel Barrymore played my grandfather. Later he played my father and finally he played my husband. If he had lived I'm sure I would have played his mother. That's the way it is in Hollywood. The men get younger and the women get older.

Lillian Gish

This isn't just food . . .

Most of us, in the tormented throes of teenage angst, will have screamed something appalling at our parents – 'I didn't ask to be born!' or something melodramatic along those lines. Many fewer of us, when parents ourselves, will have expressed the equivalent sentiment to our own children once they've become teenagers.

One of those few was Mum. She often screamed at me, 'I wish you hadn't been born!' She was usually very apologetic later on, but if pressed to be more fulsome in her apology would, like as not, claim she hadn't actually said it at all, that I'd misunderstood or (her favourite riposte) that I'd taken it the 'wrong way'. Denial was very much her style. She had wanted children, albeit more as an abstract concept and, as she once said sadly, 'so that they could love me'. But she hadn't anticipated the huge volume of drudgery and emotional turmoil that came as part of the package. I don't think she was even remotely prepared for it. Her upbringing with emotionally and physically remote parents, a nanny, and servants had certainly not afforded her the first inkling of just how mammoth a workload having children is.

For Mum one of the most onerous elements of being a mother was the weekly shop. It wasn't that she was lazy. Well, she was quite physically lazy, if by lazy you mean she'd rather read a book than go for a walk. But, really, she wasn't idle so much as irked by tasks imposed on her and especially those extra ones imposed on a mother. She didn't want to *have* to do anything at all; she resisted all routine, and none more so than the weekly shop. And she couldn't bear it when she did do it, effing and blinding as she left and more of the same when she came back, unloading the car with as much bad grace as she could muster. To be entirely fair to Mum, that's very similar to what I do now, for I loathe shopping – the only difference being that I spare my children a display of disgruntlement as part of my constant efforts to do all I can not to attach bad feelings to the provision of food.

For a brief period Mum tried to swerve the task of the weekly shop by using a cash and carry she'd stumbled upon. She'd buy stuff in bulk. For a while the cupboards housed vast tins, the size of paint cans, of powdered milk, cooking oil, hot chocolate powder, and other 'essentials'. One solitary, enormous tin of Marmite was in our kitchen for so long it ended up containing not only the hardened remains of the spread but various bits of household detritus, including, I vividly recall, more than a few pubic hairs. I can see how hair from someone's head might get trapped in a tin containing something extremely sticky, and this being the early Seventies both my older brothers sported long hair, but I never understood how someone's pubes had got in there.

When I was 15 and wanting more pocket money than Mum could provide, I got a Saturday job at Marks and Spencer's. It was about a mile away from our house, in Camden Town, the nearest high street. The day started fairly early, at about 8 a.m., and finished when the shop closed at 6 p.m. (no late opening hours in those days). I mainly worked on the till or as a shelf stacker and on a really exciting day (any variety was exciting) I might get upgraded to 'freezer checker'. For this job I'd be given a clipboard and a padded coat to protect against the cold and instructed to check the freezer (there was a clue in the job title) to ensure it was fully stocked and everything was up to date.

I really liked working there. M&S was a wonderfully caring company to work for and, with the exception of one terrifying Northern Irish supervisor, the rest of the all-female staff were friendly and chummy, despite it being glaringly obvious that I was the only middle-class person amongst them. But Bernadette, the supervisor, really had it in for me. One day, unbidden by a superior, I took it upon myself to move some Victoria sponge cakes around on the shelf. I'd noticed that the newer ones, those with dates furthest away, were in front of those with older dates, the ones we wanted to sell sooner. (When doing the weekly shop now, armed with my insider's knowledge I always take things from the back of the shelf – as if it makes a blind bit of difference.) Bernadette, a wee, dark-haired, pinch-faced hag of a woman, flew down the aisle towards me like a witch on a broomstick.

'What on earth do you think you're doing, Miss Weir?' she snapped. (Everyone was required to address each other formally. I don't know why; this was 1973, not 1934.)

'I'm rotating the stock. The newer cakes were in front of the older ones,' I replied, confident that this was a good thing and that she'd surely be pleased with me.

'And exactly who told you to do that?' she continued fiercely.

'Erm, no one. I just noticed they were the wrong way round and decided to use my own initiative.'

That was a mistake. I'd sparked her fury with my high-falutin words. She was incensed. 'Don't you *ever* use your own initiative at Marks and Spencer's!'

Duly chastened, I promised I never would again and slunk back to my till, not entirely confident that Bernadette knew what 'initiative' meant.

Much to my mother's delight, one of the best staff perks was a hefty discount on food. At the end of each Saturday any food with a sell-by date of that day or the next (a Sunday, when no shops then opened) was sold off to the staff for a tenth of the marked price. So a chicken for £1.50 (this was over 30 years ago) was 15p, a 45p cake (hey, maybe even one I'd rotated erroneously) was 4p and so on. There was often a lot of fresh produce left over and I soon got into the habit of doing what turned out to be the week's shop at the end of my day. So Mum, who hadn't yet worked out a settlement with Dad and claimed to be short of money, not only saved herself quite a bit of cash but, even more thrillingly for her, was relieved of the dreaded weekly shop. And importantly for me I was now able to ensure there'd actually be some food in the house. The fact that I'd brought the food home didn't mean I was any more entitled to eat it; no, Mum remained just as cross and controlling about it. But at least it was there to have a battle over, rather than the norm, which was that there simply wasn't any.

I never questioned whether I ought to be responsible for doing the shopping. I just did it. I often grumbled, as I trudged home after a long day at work, heaving bags laden with food. I had become the provider. There's nothing wrong with a 15-year-old helping out her mother, but I wasn't augmenting Mum's shop: I was doing it instead of her. I wasn't 'helping out': I'd become the provider. Years later, in my early thirties, I met a therapist at a party and fell into 'amusing' her with a few of the more flamboyant stories about Mum's parenting. She, taking it all in quite seriously as you might expect, said, 'Your mother made you her mother.' I thought this was a brilliant description of the ignominies to which I was subjected in my early life and couldn't wait to slap that down on the table when I next saw Mum, with a triumphant, 'Hah, how do you feel now?!' I was sure she'd be racked with shame. Here was proof from a trained psychotherapist that Mum was officially A Bad Mother. In fact, Mum's reaction was entirely typical. She broke into a broad smile, like a cheeky toddler, and said, 'Yes, and wasn't I lucky that you did! You were so good at it!'

One of the main crimes that spurred Mum into shouting at me was my poor academic performance at school. As someone who set great store by intellectual superiority (and often used hers to lord it over others foolish enough to admit in her presence that they hadn't read Chaucer in the original), she was embarrassed and annoyed by how consistently badly I did at school. I was frequently in trouble, and to make matters worse could not have cared less. Why would I have done? To fail so spectacularly was success in itself, since I was doing it on purpose. Both my parents prized being thin and being bright above all else, so what better rebellion than to make sure I was neither? Besides which, clowning around and being in trouble were how I got noticed; that was how I ensured everyone knew who I was.

After over a year of Saturdays at M&S, school suddenly became all about O-levels. To my dismay my friends began to make plans for revising at the weekends and during our spare time. Never one for going it alone and always needful of a crowd, I was immediately gripped by the conviction that I'd better join in, sure that all it would take to pass these exams was a bit of rushed, last-minute swotting. To make room for this I decided to give up my Saturday job, which was exhausting and time-consuming. You'd have thought Mum would welcome the idea; after all, she certainly wanted me to do well in my O-levels, something which would, at last, win the respect of her friends, whose children were apparently all set for double firsts at Oxbridge. But Mum went absolutely berserk. 'For Christ's sake, now I'm going to have to do the wretched bloody shopping again, you selfish girl. You only ever think about yourself.' Although Mum's irrationality was par for the course, even I was surprised.

Predictably – given that I'd done no work in the year leading up to the exams and, of course, did hardly any revision on my freed-up Saturdays – I only got two O-levels. Yet life could have been so different. When I'd handed in my notice at M&S, the manager – Bernadette's boss, who clearly recognised my retail talents (and possibly even my initiative) – tried to tempt me into staying by offering me a promotion: a permanent place as a 'freezer checker' with my own padded jacket and clipboard, quite a step up from checkout girl. I decided not to tell Mum at the time. I didn't dare. Although she'd have been very snooty about having a daughter who worked full time in a shop, she'd have been very tempted by the idea of a lifetime's supply of chicken at 15p apiece.

Actresses don't eat

At around the age of 14 I had realised I wanted to be an actress. I didn't go to the theatre all the time, I wasn't always reading plays and I wasn't part of the drama group at school. Even though Sophie and I always creatively used our bunking-off time to catch up on all the classic black-and-white movies Bette Davis had starred in, I didn't nurture unrealistic dreams of being a film star, either. I guess I just wanted to show off, to get attention, for a living, and that's what I assumed actresses did, or rather got – attention.

My parents took a very dim view of these aspirations. Mum, in particular, had typically strong and sweeping opinions about it. 'All actors are morons,' she pronounced when I told her what I wanted to be, 'except Michael Hordern. He's marvellously intelligent.' My mother didn't, of course, know Michael Hordern personally; she just assumed he was intelligent because he was such a good actor.

Her disdain for 'all actors' notwithstanding, she wasn't immune to the thrill of being in the presence of famous ones. One winter's night, Mum threw a Christmas drinks' party, to which a few of my friends were welcome. Sophie came along, having escaped from her dad and stepmother's house, which was just across the road from ours. Sophie's 'wicked' stepmother was the actress Billie Whitelaw and as neighbours she and my mother had a nodding acquaintance but weren't friends. Nonetheless that night, Billie, to Sophie's embarrassment, suddenly turned up at Mum's, having learnt there was a party and invited herself over. Billie, already a bit the worse for wear, took up a commanding position in the hallway, large glass of wine in one hand, the other running the neck-to-crotch zip on her black velour jumpsuit all the way up and down, swaying from side to side all the while, and started declaring loudly, 'I am sick and tired of being Samuel Beckett's fucking mouthpiece.' Sophie and I took refuge in the living room, howling with mortified laughter, whilst Mum and all her intellectually superior friends were starstruck. Clearly they could not get over the fact that they were in the presence of the greatest British theatre actress of the day and, what was more, the muse of one of the world's greatest playwrights. Never mind that she was drunk and not behaving brilliantly: she was famous and iconic plays had been written *for* her by Samuel Beckett, no less!

Aspiring to be an actress when you know yourself to be fat, or at the very least unconventionally shaped, is a strange ambition. Especially in 1971, when there were no fat women on television. There were very few women on television at all, and those few were, without exception, beautiful, sexy, slim, and playing second banana to male actors, who were, predictably enough, much more representative of the ordinary range of men-in-the-street.

Actually, there was one fat woman on telly when I decided I wanted to be an actress: Hattie Jacques. She was a very large, not particularly pretty woman who always played sour-faced harridans (most notably Matron in the *Carry on* films). Her character inevitably had a scene in which she, wearing something comically flimsy (i.e. inappropriate for someone that large), would attempt to have sex with an unwilling man. The clear message – even to the teenage me, not looking for subtext – was that he was unwilling because she was fat, ugly, and randy. Of course he didn't want to have sex with her!

Nevertheless, with only Hattie Jacques as my guide (as it were), I set my sights on becoming an actress. So crazy does that sound to me now that it seems like aspiring to be an astronaut when you're afraid of the dark, or a professional skier when you've got no legs. I don't know what I was thinking, but evidently I was fired up by the prospect of conquering something that gave every indication of being unconquerable by me. There I was, believing that I was going to conquer it, come what may. I was going to *make* it like me.

Leaving school, I failed to get into every single drama school of my choice (perhaps I ought to have taken that as a sign) and ended up training at a dismal, insignificant college which mainly focused on the academic side of acting (is there one?). I left there with a diploma in performance arts (so useful) but still lacking focus and direction and, for want of anything else to do, threw myself into getting an acting job.

Once I started auditioning – a hideously humiliating process for anyone, irrespective of their looks – I quickly discovered that I really wasn't equipped with any of the essential attributes needed to make it as an actress: a great figure, an unusually attractive face, and a winning personality. In fact, quite the opposite: as a plump, fairly stroppy, and not particularly pretty girl, what I was actually equipped for was instant rejection. And that's pretty much what I got, nine times out of ten.

When I started out in 1979, the other actresses of my age who, like me, sat in waiting room after waiting room were girls like Joanne Whalley, Phoebe Nicholls, and Greta Scacchi. And even when it wasn't them specifically, my contemporaries and competitors were gorgeous, slim, confident girls with (as I saw it) the world at their feet. They were all so slim that if you'd bunched them all up together, they'd still have weighed less than I did at the time. Now, of course, one might think it a bit odd that I – who was unlike all those actresses in every possible way – was going up for the same parts as them; but that's just how it works. Unless the part actually specifies that the actress should have brown hair, blue eyes, or two heads, directors are usually happy to meet a variety of actresses in the hope that one will jump out at them, figuratively speaking, as perfect for the part.

In those days, however, it was never the fat one. I know now that I should never have put myself through the torture of competing with those girls – but that's the luxury of hindsight. My agent got me the auditions, so off I went. I certainly didn't have enough self-knowledge or self-confidence to judge whether or not I was right for the part. The vast majority of actors, male and female, are so desperate for an acting job, any acting job, that there's no room to work out whether you're right for the job, the statistical likelihood of getting it or the merits of the job itself. You already live hand to mouth, in a hugely competitive arena within which you strongly (and rightly) suspect that your individual merit has little to do with your chances of employment. If you're lucky, the one thing you have going for you is that *you* believe you're great, but until someone else does, too (and you're the one who has to convince them of your greatness) you're just an out-of-work actor. (And I didn't even have that. In fact, I suspected I was a bit shit.) It's hardly likely that this competitive world is going to foster an atmosphere in which you'll be able to develop a considered and measured approach to auditions.

So there I was in the waiting room, perched nervously on an unforgivingly hard-to-get-up-from sofa, wearing a Liberty-print dress or a flowery skirt and 'peasant' blouse (this was the late Seventies) – whatever it was, something flowing and chosen specifically to flatter and cover my 'sins'. Whatever it was had been analysed, discussed (if there was anyone around prepared to discuss it), and painstakingly picked out over a period of at least two hours (there was nothing else to do all day except prepare for these wretched auditions), with the express intention of hiding my fat arse, flabby arms, and loose stomach. When I saw the other actresses in the room, sitting there casually wearing tight jeans and equally tight tops, or tiny dresses, or just ordinary nothing-to-hide outfits, as well they might, I immediately realised that, compared to them, I looked like an elephant wearing a sofa cover designed for a smaller elephant. It took years before I realised that putting me up against those girls was laughable – cruel even. But we were the same age, and on paper I ought to have had a chance; there were no rules stating that plump girls didn't get a look-in. That's just the way it shook down; no one actually wrote a manifesto stating there was no place for us on television or anywhere else. If only they had, then we'd have known where we stood and belonged: on the outside looking in.

Even when I did well in auditions, I was often asked if I'd lose weight, but never for a specific reason – never because the part was for a girl who hadn't eaten for a year or had a wasting disease or was being held in a prisoner-of-war camp. I remember one director in particular (I don't know why, because this incident was pretty much how most of the auditions went). He was in his mid-forties, and no oil painting himself, it has to be said. As I left the room he sidled up to me and said, 'You're a pretty girl, but you could lose some weight. You're a bit too fat, really.'

Now, it's outrageous that he said that, but then and there I didn't feel outrage. I just smiled pleasantly and nodded in agreement. A minuscule bit of me wanted to say, 'Too fat for what, exactly?' I wanted to challenge him to expand on what he meant and his justification for saying it. There was a tiny, as yet unformed, bit of me thinking, Surely this is wrong. But there was a much bigger bit of me, conditioned by years of disapproval and never-ending exposure to fantasy images of how a girl 'ought' to look, that won every time (just not enough to lose weight). That bit of me desperately wanted the job, wanted the approval and validation the job would represent, and was certainly prepared to agree that I was indeed too fat, not just for this part but for life as a whole.

Of course there were times when a director recognised my potential, though on occasion not for the job for which I'd auditioned. A couple of experiences spring to mind. Theatres putting on big productions of musicals used to hold 'open calls', which were basically one mass audition. An announcement would appear in the *Stage*, the actors' trade paper, giving the name of a production, an address, and a date and time, calling for 'actors and dancers who can sing'. It really was as non-specific as that. So, naturally, the entire world would turn up. You'd queue around the block in the freezing cold for hours, waiting to be seen. Eventually, you'd be invited to enter the theatre and give your name and details, before walking out on to the sparsely lit stage to face an almost empty auditorium where a handful of people – usually a director, choreographer, musical director, casting director, and maybe a few assistants – would be staring up at you. This group might, if you were lucky, greet you with a quick hello, but more than likely you'd get just a cursory nod of acknowledgement followed by an invitation to sing something and maybe dance around a bit.

On one of the many occasions I put myself through this excruciating experience I auditioned for a part in the chorus of *The Best Little Whorehouse in Texas* (a musical whose title gives an admirably concise picture of what the show's about). I wore a suitably low-cut top, revealing what I hoped was an attractive yet not-too-tarty cleavage, and a tight belt over a voluminous skirt – all suggesting, I hoped, a 'saucy' look that indicated I'd be perfect for this job. I thought I might have a chance at this one, actually, since I reasoned there were surely 'curvy' girls keeping the cowboys company in the American Midwest.

At the end of my song the director stood up and said, 'Thank you. Can you wait at the side? I'd like to talk to you.'

I'd caught his attention. The ghastly, humiliating process had paid off. Things were looking up. I was thrilled. As requested, I found a corner of the wings offstage and waited for the director.

When he appeared he was smiling kindly, hand outstretched. 'That was great – thanks! Erm, there's nothing for you in this show, but I wondered if you'd be interested in being in *Winnie the Pooh*, a kids' production I'm doing for primary schools soon?' *Winnie the Pooh*?! I'd done myself up like a dog's dinner to get the part of a Texan tart, but all he saw was my suitability for the part of a honey-addicted tubby bear. 'We'd give you a costume,' he added helpfully, presumably taking my stunned expression as concern that I might not resemble the bear closely enough to do the part justice.

On another ill-fated occasion I actually managed to turn down a part. It was to be in a year-long tour of the stage version of *The Seven Year Itch*, starring Patrick Mower and Una Stubbs, if you please, in the part immortalised on screen by Marilyn Monroe. I was offered the part of a girl who appears in the lead actor's fantasy. She wears nothing but a baby-doll nightie and doesn't speak. I had been out of work for a whole year, but even so I just couldn't do it, much as I needed the work and the money. But I got a call from the producer, an American man in his late seventies. (My agent, who was urging me to accept the job, had helpfully given him my home number.) 'Listen,' he said brusquely, 'I know what the problem is.' I was surprised. How could this guy have worked out that I thought the part and the show were rubbish? He was putting money into it; surely he, at least, must think it was good? 'I know what it is, but it's OK. We think you're a very pretty girl, so don't worry about the fat legs. We can hide them easily enough with the right nightie.' As far as he was concerned, that *must* have been the problem – what else could it possibly be?

Of course, if (as I did back then) you spent time with actresses, particularly successful ones, you would find that in fact they didn't eat. So here was another solid reason to equate success with being thin, and moreover caring enough about success to stay thin by not eating. A year after I'd started acting Karel gave me a very small part in his new movie, *The French Lieutenant's Woman*, starring a rising American star, Meryl Streep. I'd seen her in *Kramer vs Kramer* but, other than that, knew little of her. Notwithstanding the huge chasm between our statuses in the movie, because of my friendship with the Reiszs most days on the shoot I'd have lunch with Betsy, Karel, and Meryl, who was friendly and put me at my ease. Even though she'd just had her first child, all she had for lunch every day was an apple and a small slice of cheese. I was filled with admiration and envy of her commitment to keeping her figure and her ability to master her hunger (she *had* to be hungry, surely).

She wasn't just turning in a great performance (and, what's more, in an English accent): she was on 24-hour figure-watch, too. She was multi-tasking big time, and with the things that mattered. She deserved to be successful.

I didn't. I was on 24-hour eating-the-bacon-rolls that were constantly served up by the location caterers.

The belief that there's a correlation between success and thinness, and similarly that abstinence equates with just deserts (rather than desserts), is widespread; but it's writ super-large, for all to see, in the world of actresses. Twenty years later, this skewed view of how an actress ought to look still prevailed. In 1998, a review in the *Guardian* newspaper of the film *Titanic* said of Kate Winslet: 'And she is – sorry to have to say this, but there's no other way – too fleshy to be convincing either as her mother's daughter or as someone Dawson would fall for.' So Richard Williams, the reviewer, thought not only that she was too fat to be someone's daughter (do only fat people have fat children?) but that she was too fat to be loved by someone as beautiful and (one assumes) thin as Leonardo DiCaprio (playing Dawson)? And this was the *Guardian* – let's not forget, a highbrow left-leaning newspaper – not the *Sun* or *Hello!*, where one might expect to read nasty comments about an actress's weight as if they related to her acting ability.

During those largely bleak and unsuccessful years of auditions, so delusional and desperate was I that there'd be times when I'd just lie outright to get a job. In 1984, I auditioned for a season of plays in Musselburgh, just outside Edinburgh. The three plays were to be a music-hall rendition of the story of Dr Crippen, an Agatha Christie-style whodunnit and *The Prime of Miss Jean Brodie.* To my surprise, the audition went rather well – surely, I thought in that instant, thanks to the fact that I'd recently lost some weight. Couldn't be anything else, after all. Of course, I knew I was still fat; but the few pounds I'd lost, combined with some clever dressing, had allowed me to con this director into thinking I was thinner that I really was. As we parted company, the director offered me the job. I didn't really want to spend four months in a not-very-prestigious theatre in a bleak, wind-battered East Lothian town, but all the same I was thrilled, naturally.

As we said our goodbyes, my new employer coughed and looked a little uneasy. '. . . And you're OK with the nude scene in *Miss Jean Brodie*, yeah?'

'Erm . . .' I replied, wetly, playing for time. I'd seen the film, but ages ago, and couldn't think what he was talking about. 'The scene where Sandy, that's your part, poses naked for the art teacher. It's what the drama of the whole play hinges on. You're OK with that?'

My head spun. I couldn't take it in. Naked? On stage, in front of strangers, with-no-clothes-on-at-all naked? Did he mean *that* kind of naked? How could he have known that he was asking me to face my very worst fear? So incredibly lacking in the confidence required to appear naked in front of anyone was I that his chances of my offering him a quick blow-job there and then were far higher than getting me to say yes to this. Good God, I couldn't even appear naked in front of myself, let alone a theatre filled with strangers. I couldn't believe my appalling luck. Here I was being offered four months' work, after ages of miserable, boring, endless unemployment, and it all hinged on one sodding scene in one play. It was just too awful.

So what did I do? Did I listen to my inner voice, the voice that knew me well, screaming 'No, not naked! Anything but naked!' Of course not. I did what any actress would do who has dressed cleverly enough to disguise the fact that she's actually 'too fat' to appear naked, but now has to reap what she's sown because the disguise has worked. 'Yeah, sure, that's not a problem,' I said, knowing even as the words stumbled their way out of my mouth that the day would never dawn when I WOULD BE NAKED ON STAGE – not for one nanosecond, never mind a whole scene. It was all my own fault: if I hadn't tricked him with my outfit, then he'd have seen how fat I really was and never offered me the job in the first place, never mind asked me to take my clothes off, too. It wasn't his fault. He couldn't possibly know how disgusting I looked in the nude. He couldn't begin to guess just how revolting my tits were, how fat my stomach was, how wobbly and huge my arse was, when they were all unclothed. I'd done a little fan dance, all smoke and mirrors, and he'd bought it. I'd managed to pretend, for 20 or so minutes, that I was the kind of girl someone might want to see in the nude, and *now* look what had happened. I was going to have to pay for the deception.

As I made my way back to the Tube station in a trance I thought about what I'd done. I knew I'd agreed to appear naked on stage in about a month's time. But I also knew, deep down, that that was never, ever going to happen. I was stuck.

Soon enough, deep in denial, up I duly went to Scotland to start the season, weighed down all the while by the imminent not-going-to-happen nudity. It was just like having a dead body hidden in my trunk, only not as smelly. The stint started with the Crippen play, and all went well. Yet as each day passed and the rehearsals for *Miss Brodie* drew closer, I dreamt of contracting a debilitating illness or uniquely placed rash that would suddenly, through no fault of my own, mean I couldn't actually appear completely naked in the play.

Then, out of the blue, the gods smiled on me. There had been some protests, and the local council decided that the theatre, which it funded, should not mount *The Prime of Miss Jean Brodie* after all. The reason? Well, it was the nude scene. The protest was not, from what I gathered, a campaign against the horror of seeing me, specifically, in the nude; it was against nudity per se (this being provincial Scotland in the early Eighties). The fact that the audience was to be spared the sight of me naked was just a fortuitous side issue for them and me. Since the whole play hinges on that scene, it was eventually decided that it would be better to put on something better tailored to local sensibilities. So, thanks to people very much like my Granny She-She, I was saved – or rather, they were. To this day I have absolutely no idea what I'd have done if the perceived delicacy of the residents of East Lothian hadn't intervened. I'd probably have made sure I got that rash, come hell or high water.

I persevered with this unfriendly career not because I had a burning desire to act, nor because I knew, despite all the rejections, I was brilliant – *au contraire*. I kept on going because I had absolutely no idea what else to do. That and because I was aware that I felt alive (and loved) when 'mucking about' or showing off, as it might more accurately be described, and acting seemed like the closest thing.

By choosing acting as a career, what I really did was choose a job which, given all the evidence available, was likely to be a self-fulfilling prophecy, a stick with which to beat myself. It was going to reject me, confirming what I already believed: that I was too fat to succeed. On the few occasions when I did manage to drop a bit of weight, I was bewildered when I didn't get the parts any more easily than when I'd been fatter. It wasn't until I found out what I was good at that work began to pick up. While my weight did affect my employability (and always would have done), the ultimate barrier to employment was that I was trying to be something I wasn't. I wasted all that time trying for roles that were only ever going to go to thin beauties. All that time being a square peg in a round hole (well, more of a round peg in a square hole).

Doctor No

With my out-of-work-actress days either filled by going to auditions with other much thinner actresses, or empty with acres and acres of time to think about what was wrong with me, I had ample opportunity to notice how fat I was. I'd always felt fat, but once I became an actress I had an added reason to chart my size daily, sometimes hourly.

As I've said, there weren't any fat actresses out there, so I couldn't have been cast as one. Anyway, even at my heaviest I was never big enough to qualify for Hattie-Jacques-type parts, had they been on offer. It's difficult to give you an accurate, objective picture of exactly how fat I was – probably a size 16, but depending on my moods I fluctuated from feeling OK to feeling enormous. Fat, for most of us, is mainly a state of mind. I definitely wasn't Hattie-size; even I, in my bleakest I'll-never-get-a-job moments, knew that. But I absolutely *definitely* wasn't thin. I was sort of ... well, me-shaped, with a bum that was disproportionately big for the rest of my body.

That made it quite easy, if I dressed judiciously, to con people into believing that I wasn't actually fat, so long as they didn't see me in the nude. Since I could take it for granted that only people who were already keen on me would ever see me naked (and even then, as we've established, never standing up), I thought I had all the bases covered. And I very rarely wore trousers since they, more than most items of clothing, highlighted my *bête noire* – the fat arse. However, cleverly camouflaging my 'problem areas' sometimes meant I landed myself in a worse situation than if I'd gone out and proud in, for example, tight jeans.

Naturally enough, I guess, with too much time on my hands and nothing very real to occupy my waking hours, the more and more I minded about being overweight the more weight I ended up putting on. Eventually, I talked it through with my GP who, learning that my periods were irregular, thought I might be suffering from some genuine medical condition such as an underactive thyroid, and referred me to a consultant.

After a few weeks' wait, I was given an appointment. Dressed in my best 'I'm not that fat' outfit, I went off to the hospital. There I was met by the consultant, a surprisingly good-looking guy who, I guessed, was about 30 or so. We hit it off straight away. He was friendly, jokey, and I'd go as far as to say flirty. I was pretty sure he fancied me, but immediately worried this could only be because I was wearing my 'thin' clothes and he hadn't realised how fat I actually was.

However, his demeanour soon dispelled my anxiety. He listened patiently as I explained to him that, as an actress,

I was 'too fat' and ought to be thin. In response, he embarked on a long, heartening, and politically sound discussion of what 'too fat' actually meant. I was enthralled, and encouraged that, instead of seeing me as a medical case, he was engaging with what he described as my 'skewed vision' of the world. Warming to his theme, he suggested I celebrate the fact that, in his medical opinion, I had the constitution of a 'famine survivor' – someone built to last. He explained that a famine survivor, given exactly the same daily ration of calories as someone with a less efficient physiology, would stay alive much longer. He really wanted me to see how mixed up my thinking was. In the seventeenth century, he said, a figure like mine would have been the pinnacle of fashion, a desirable demonstration that I was wealthy, healthy, and most unlikely ever to succumb to poverty-induced starvation.

I was flattered that he was putting so much effort into convincing me that, as he saw it, I was wasting my time focusing needlessly on an issue that wasn't real. The sensible, intelligent part of me appreciated his argument, wanting to believe that, of course, it was only in the shallow world of acting that people like me – who were, after all, only a bit plump – were 'too fat'.

Meanwhile, the other, desperate-to-conform-and-thereby-succeed part of me, the part in the driving seat, was thinking, This is all very well if I were pursuing a career in, say, teaching, but I *want* to be an actress, and, sound as his point of view may be, it won't hold much sway in the world I've chosen. I also couldn't help noticing that, as we weren't actually in the seventeenth century, it was of scant use to me to find out I'd still be going strong when all my serfs had kicked the bucket. I lamely tried to set up a counter-argument but it wasn't easy, given that I didn't really understand why all actresses had to be the same tiny size. I just desperately wanted to be a successful actress, and I wanted him to help by making me thinner.

All the same, I really warmed to him. I was deeply touched, and grateful to him for putting so much effort into convincing me that real women came in all shapes and sizes, and that the world was a better place for that. But, more than anything, I still wanted to be thinner – and I told him so, clinging to the hope that I might turn out to have a condition for which he'd prescribe some magic pills that would help me achieve my goal. So he took my medical history and said he'd do a quick examination, 'just in case there is anything physically awry'. I should go into his exam room and take off my clothes, he said, while he fetched a female nurse.

Having had such a comforting and reassuring discussion with him about women's bodies, I had no qualms about doing so. I'd found him to be an intelligent, kind person who'd made it abundantly clear that he understood that I wasn't a greedy pig who stuffed her face all day long; rather, as he'd told me, my body stored food much more readily than it burnt it off.

I waited, naked except for my knickers. When he came back, accompanied by a young, slim nurse, I noticed that he shot me a quick, slightly puzzled look. As he reached for a pair of surgical gloves, he glanced over at me again. There was a short, sharp intake of breath; then he crinkled up his nose as if he'd just caught a whiff of some awful smell, and said, 'Actually, you know, you could lose a pound or two.'

I thought I was going to die of shame. Instantly, my naked fatness filled the room, blubber wobbling and pulsating into every nook and cranny. For a blissful half-hour, my self-consciousness about my size had ebbed under the warm glow of his morale-boosting proselytising. Now, as if ignited by his disappointed expression, I'd exploded into the fattest person in the world.

I'd like to tell you that the nurse and I exchanged sisters-under-the-skin expressions of outrage. I'd like to tell you that I jumped up, grabbed his stethoscope, and stuffed it down his throat. I'd like to tell you that he immediately realised what he'd said and apologised. But I can't. I just sat there as he poked and prodded me for a few minutes, while tears of shame prickled my eyes. 'No, I don't think there's anything medically wrong. You just need to diet if you want to lose weight,' he casually announced.

I left feeling much, much fatter (and more miserable, naturally) than when I'd arrived. What's more, I knew it was all my fault. He wasn't to blame. He hadn't intended to humiliate me. I'd led him up the garden path by wearing my cleverly swirly 'I'm not really fat at all' skirt, instead of my 'see how fat I really am' jeans. An important, busy consultant like him would never have wasted his time preaching all that feminist stuff had he known how fat I really was. All that great stuff was intended for someone he found attractive, and I'd disappointed him. It wasn't for a girl who, in the nude, actually *was* fat, and was therefore unqualified to be fancied by special, clever him.

I walked away feeling that I'd asked for this, that I *ought* to have looked fatter from the start. I should have worn my fatness on my sleeve and then he'd never have been compelled to put me in my place like that. He was obviously humiliated that I'd tricked him into finding me attractive – which he clearly had, until he'd caught sight of my rolls of fat cascading unattractively over the top of my knickers like a slow-motion avalanche of cake mixture.

I was furious, too, and indignant. However, as yet, I didn't have the confidence to translate that into asking him what had happened to his 'famine survivor' argument, so convincingly constructed only a few minutes earlier. I didn't ask him if my newly revealed fat was a health risk. I didn't ask him if he thought his remark was appropriate, sensitive, or in any way, shape, or form supportive and helpful. I didn't have the wherewithal, the sense of righteousness to ask him what he thought the odds were on him staying alive long enough to celebrate his next birthday if he carried on talking like that to women with body-image issues. I didn't begin to think he might be in the wrong.

Some ladies smoke too much
and some ladies drink too much
and some ladies pray too much.
But all ladies think that they weigh
too much.

'Curl up and Diet' from *Candy is Dandy:
The Best of Ogden Nash* by Ogden Nash

Allergies for attention

I moved out of the family home in my early twenties but for long after (in fact, always) I'd left Mum's house I still dreaded going there if any eating was to be done. I knew no visit involving consumption would ever pass without her drawing attention to my eating – whatsoever. Mum liked a drink accompanied by a bowl of nuts or crisps, and although we often had nice evenings chatting over a bottle of wine, not one of them, ever, was free of comment. When I reached for the snacks, she simply could not help herself. As I took a handful she'd suck her breath in sharply, as if she'd just witnessed a horrific accident, lean theatrically forward, pick up the bowl very slowly, and move it to just out of my reach, exclaiming, 'Watching you eat nuts is like having hot pins stuck into my eyes. They're so fattening, darling, it's agony for me to see you stuffing your face with them.' (Mum was very flamboyant. Apparently, it wasn't just that I was not caring about the huge number of calories I was consuming, but to make matters worse, I was scoffing them like a starving medieval peasant.)

She always put the snacks out but never wanted me to eat them. How the evening progressed depended entirely on how robust I was feeling. If I felt cheerful I'd bat these comments back and move forward. But if I rose to the bait and responded rationally with something like, 'Why do you put them out if I'm not allowed to eat them?', Mum and I would be in for a big row.

We went through this rigmarole every single time she was at the helm – alone or with others present. Like as not, when there were more people around they'd laugh at Mum's antics and she loved it. This was sport to her and, I have to confess, very funny to witness – I can see that. But it was absolutely infuriating for me and although I learnt to make a joke of it, usually, it was a constant source of irritation for me and therefore something Mum never stopped doing.

As the years went by and Mum got older she became if not softer, and certainly not more indulgent as a mother, then much less depressed and more fun to be around. I was living in a flat and was therefore now able to go it alone and beat myself up about eating and being fat without my mother's constant, erm, help. As time went by and I got some distance from Mum, I was able to appreciate her great qualities and how difficult life had been for her as a young mother and unhappy wife. Even though, almost to her dying day, she remained capable of driving me completely round the bend, especially with food-related nagging, she became very good at being teased. You could send Mum up mercilessly and, in the main, she'd take it in the spirit it was meant and end up laughing until she cried. It was at times like these that Mum was at her best – lively, witty, and entertaining. One of us, really, more than she was a mother figure. She loved being the centre of attention, and would probably have been a much happier person had she been brought up with brothers and sisters and all the teasing that goes hand in hand with having siblings.

If you like being the centre of attention there is, of course, a constant need for an audience to provide that attention. As Mum got older and lost interest in dinner parties, at which she'd always been the queen bee, whether she was hosting the dinner or not, she turned to discovering new ailments from which she could imagine she was suffering. She was also, I suspect, a bit lonely and not busy enough, either – a killer combination, and I'm sure the reason many people resort to seeking out 'experts' who will tell them categorically how things are supposed to be. A prime example of this would be a life coach. Mercifully, Mum never quite went as far as paying one of them to tell her how to 'maximise her potential' but she did visit a woman who practised the 'art' of Colour Me Beautiful. After parting with nearly £100 Mum found out that she didn't suit acid yellow or lime green. Mmm, what a surprise. Few of us do. She went through a phase of visiting various specialists to find out what was 'wrong' with her. Not that there was ever anything manifestly wrong with Mum, who had a strong constitution and was astonishingly brave for someone so self-indulgent in other ways. (When she was in her mid-sixties, she woke up one night to find a teenage drug addict ransacking her bedroom. He threatened to kill her if she didn't keep quiet. 'No you bloody well won't!' she told him. 'This is my house, and I won't be spoken to like that. And if you were going to kill me you'd already have done it.' He escaped with her jewellery, but he didn't kill her. Thanks to her years in teaching, Mum later explained, she was immune to the empty threats of 'cross boys'.) In fact, when Mum was properly ill towards the end of her life she had no interest in and put no effort into finding out what was wrong with her.

One of the specialists upon whom Mum happily lit was a food allergist. Oh, happy day for her (and him) when those two met. Now, real allergies exist, I know. For example, the lips of one of the teachers at my kids' school turn bright red and swell up like a couple of inner tyres if she so much as walks past an apple, a plum, or a pear – odd, but true. One of my best friends is instantly covered in a nasty rash, from head to toe, if she applies sun cream. Fair enough. These are allergies. They have been discovered by a process of elimination after an immediate and serious, or at the very least mightily uncomfortable, reaction to the offending allergens. They do not generally come to light as a result of boredom, self-centred idleness, and having too much disposable income. Unless you *believe*.

The only otherwise-fighting-fit people I know who have 'discovered' allergies have done so following visits to ludicrously expensive 'allergy specialists' (who often, it turns out, are also skilled crystal readers, homeopaths, and chakra merchants). These people have not discovered these allergies after a nasty physical reaction to a particular substance, nor in response to repeated, inexplicable bouts of rashes, bumps, or watering eyes. Someone else has *told* them that they are allergic to something which, up until that moment, hasn't bothered them one bit. That's a bit like being told you're pregnant when you haven't had sex – surely you'd know because it'd be happening to you and you'd do something about it, not the other way round.

Yet when my mother in her seventies and feeling a little lethargic (at that age you would, wouldn't you?) went to see the highly recommended (by whom remains a mystery) Dr Kostalides – an 'expert' in ... can't remember exactly what (charging too much money and not much else, as far as my siblings and I could make out), she proclaimed that he was the answer to all her prayers. For £75 an hour (oh yes) he informed Mum that she was allergic to wheat and wine and henceforward must eschew all wheat-based products and drink only champagne. I'm not sure how champagne qualifies as not wine, but there you go: I'm not a 'healer'.

He'd given Mum exactly what she was looking for: attention and the licence to be a demanding pain in the arse at mealtimes, and an expensive one at that. Having made his pronouncement, he said he had to see her a few more times. Of course he'd need to see her again.

Fresh from her second visit, Mum was full of the joys of spring. 'Oh, he was wonderful, darlings, so knowledgeable, so in tune with me from the moment he set eyes on me.'

My sister Christina and I, who had arranged our visits to the house to coincide with each other, exchanged weary looks.

'He knew I was wheat intolerant before he'd even examined me. He could tell from the moment I walked into the room.'

The temptation was too great for me. 'So how does he think you managed to get to the ripe old age of 74 eating all that bread, then?'

'I knew *you'd* be sarcastic about this, but I don't care. I feel so much better since I started seeing him.'

'Well, most people feel better when they stop eating bread, or any other major food group which has made up a disproportionate amount of their daily diet,' Christina said in a matter-of-fact voice. She then produced an assortment of delicious sandwiches she'd picked up en route, for our lunch. She shot me a mischievous look as she laid them out on a plate. We both knew what was coming. Mum licked her lips and gingerly extended a hand towards the plate.

'I think you'll find that sandwiches are made with bread . . .' Christina said in her most innocent tone of voice.

'Which, I believe, is made of wheat . . .' I added.

'And we don't want you to have an anaphylactic shock, do we, Mum?' Christina continued.

Mum knew the game was up. 'Oh, fuck off, the pair of you. I'm hungry. He pays me attention and that's what I like,' she snapped, grabbing one half of an avocado, chicken, and mayonnaise on granary bread.

'Even if it costs you £75 an hour?' I asked.

'Yes,' she replied defiantly, chomping happily on her sandwich.

'Fine,' said my sister. 'I think from now on we'll call Dr Kostalides Dr Cost-a-lot,' by which name he was known, to us at least, for as long as Mum continued to see him. And while she was in his thrall she wouldn't go so far as to admit he was a charlatan.

Mum carried on seeing him until she got bored, and until it was clear that she hadn't turned into the new person she'd anticipated she'd be, despite the occasional bout of not eating bread and drinking only champagne. His sessions, phoney or not, had offered her individual attention, with the added allure of a 'new her' for extra piquancy and irresistibility. And when that didn't happen she lost interest.

Despite his amazing 'discoveries', Mum managed to live until the day before her eighty third birthday, having gone back to drinking wine and eating bread with gay abandon and indeed impunity. So, notwithstanding Mum's considerable intelligence, she, like many of us today searching for 'answers' rather than personal responsibility for our actions, had fallen prey to the con of modern chicanery, masquerading as new medicine. A made-up set of 'commandments' to help us kid ourselves that if we're overweight, it couldn't *possibly* be that we just eat and drink too much.

The appeal of obliteration

Like most young people, I imagine, as I got older and began to think more about what life would be like when I was an adult (and by adult, I mean when I had a job and a flat), I was unswervingly confident that I would feel, and be, grown-up. And 'grown-up', in my mind, was very different from being 'young'. I was fairly self-destructive when I was young – I couldn't seem to stop myself – but I was sure I wouldn't be like that once I'd grown up, once I was mature.

I was aware that many of the adults of my acquaintance, my parents' friends or my friends' parents, some with jobs, all with houses or flats, weren't very grown-up. After all, nearly every one of them was divorced, drank too much at parties and started crying or shouting, moaned about work, and yelled at their kids; some of the male ones even tried flirting with my friends and me (inappropriate and yuck) – all in all not very grown-up behaviour to me. But that, I decided, was because they were all fucked-up, rather than grown-up. There was something wrong with them, their lives were flawed. And obviously nothing was going to be 'wrong' with me. I felt flawed, too, but I was sure I'd be less flawed, better, when I was older. I wasn't going to be damaged, like those adults were. I wasn't going to be divorced, bitter, pissed off, stuck in a job I hated. If bad things happened to me I'd get over them, fix them, leave them. In my view, back then, proper grown-ups weren't entitled to be weak, to display their failures; they weren't allowed to be faulty.

But here I now am, undeniably older, and it turns out I'm flawed, too! I'm still surprised when I drink so much that I end up being sick. Or eat so much that I feel bloated and ill. That was what I did when I was young. Younger Me was sure that Older Me wasn't going to do that sort of thing. I was sure that proper, mature grown-ups didn't. Yet grown-up me does. I was sure self-restraint came as standard in the Grown-Up Package. I'm not saying it happens all the time these days, but I must confess that I'm still quite likely to drink a whole bottle of wine or eat all of a large bar of chocolate, only then to wonder what on earth I've done – sometimes even in the moment, while I'm actually pouring the fourth glass or wolfing down the tenth chunk. I'm out of control in those moments. The rest of the time I am fairly adult: I exercise regularly, I answer my correspondence, household bills are paid on time, dentists' visits are arranged, the kids are never late for school and always have their PE kits on the appointed days. But I regularly, wantonly seek out obliteration. Why?

Much as I now wish I hadn't gorged myself on boys and food quite as much as I did, there is no denying that there's something very seductive about overindulgence. When (and if) you revisit each individual gorgefest and pick it apart with the question 'Was it worth it?' it doesn't usually stand up to scrutiny. In fact, with the distance of time it seems unbelievable that you did it in the first place, given your armoury of understanding of the ills of drinking and eating too much. But that doesn't allow for the feeling you're having in the moment of gorging – and it's one of the best.

The first time I got so drunk I couldn't stand up was when I was 15 years old. Friday and Saturday nights, without fail, my friends and I would head down to a large pub with a huge garden on the edge of the lower reaches of Hampstead Heath. I don't know who set up the rendezvous originally but it was a fixture, and the place where all the boys we liked from various different schools would gather to indulge in under-age drinking. In those days all the teenagers I knew could get served in pubs. It seems to be harder now, or maybe people are less well disposed to indulging teenagers than they were in the Seventies. Then, the landlord certainly knew we were all under age, but he didn't seem to care, especially as we were providing good custom.

This was long before pubs had been turned into middle-class watering holes. This public house was simply an unremarkable, not very attractive north London pub. Now, it would be listed in fashionable magazines for its award-winning eaterie and esoteric wine list, but back then it was beer for the boys and shorts or lager for the girls. I was drinking vodka gimlets (essentially vodka and lime) – a surprising drink, I now think, perhaps even a bit of a pretentious, ooh-look-at-me beverage. (My interest in it had been piqued by an early obsession with the books of Raymond Chandler, in which his lead character, Philip Marlowe, always drank a gimlet.) And on this particular night I just kept going.

Various boys bought me drinks and I must have bought several myself. My gang from school, including Sophie and Sue, would always go to the pub together. Yet somehow no one ever got as drunk as me. Either I bought more, or I got boys to buy me extra drinks – very likely, since 'getting' boys to do things for me was *the* key means I had of testing (or rather proving, for that's what it was all about) my current popularity rating.

In this first episode of a series that was going to run off and on for the rest of my life, I drank so much that when it was time to go home I staggered out of the pub, got a few yards down the road, fell down, and begged to be left there on the pavement to sleep. 'I'll be fine, I'll be fine,' I insisted slurrily. It's my good fortune that Sue and Sophie refused to take me at my word and kept tugging at my arm to get me up off the floor. Others from my gang would quite happily have left me there, I'm sure. One in particular, the girl who'd marvelled when Nick had chosen me when she was available, was always very steely, and she thought my behaviour disgusting and 'unattractive'. This girl had very firm (and evidently very successful) ideas on what girls did and did not do in front of boys. Letting them see you on the loo was out; eating at all in their presence was a no-no ('you mustn't talk about being hungry in front of boys,' she announced haughtily one day and, as she was the only one thus far who'd lost her virginity, we took her at her word); and getting so pissed you tried to lie down in the street was a big faux pas. Eventually, somehow, I was got home. On those nights we didn't calorie count since we weren't eating, just drinking, and anyway in those day no one talked about the calorific value of alcohol – no one had heard of empty calories.

I tell this story not because it's unusual, least of all for an urban teenager, but because these episodes – of drinking too much and eating too much – still happen in my life. (I say 'happen'. Accidents happen; drinking or eating far too much doesn't 'happen'. So I should say, 'I still do this.' Not the sleeping in the street bit, but that's only because I'm not out late at night on my own these days.)

And how on earth can I still be doing this in my fifties? What am I after? The answer can only be obliteration. Obliteration is a place where I haven't got any responsibilities, and that makes it very appealing. Given that there's no intoxicating element to overeating, that particular form of obliteration doesn't help me blot out all of life's burdens. But it is a space where I don't have to think about anything else apart from stuffing myself. It's a place where I'm deliberately *not* thinking about what I'm doing. When I'm overeating I'm very much not watching what I eat. I'm aggressively not doing that. I've spent a *lifetime* doing that, but in those moments I'm sliding down the self-control mountain at full speed shouting 'Wheeeeeeee!' and doing what I like. I'm aware, if such a thing is possible, that I'm eating to excess defiantly, on purpose, in spite of not wanting more. I'm hurting myself, I guess, because obviously I'm not hurting anyone else by eating too much. I guess I might be hurting my parents retrospectively, paying them back for all the years of controlling my eating – unresolved as that may seem.

And when it's drink, there is, apparently, no cut-off mechanism, no ability to tell my already inebriated self that it's time to stop because, if I don't, the next stage will be vomiting, a crippling headache, and falling asleep wherever I may be.

The most uncomfortable aspect of this kind of obliteration is that it sets up those around you, in the moment, as the 'carer'. Those of us who overindulge make the people close to us take charge, whether they like it or not, by rendering ourselves incapacitated. For example, last night I rang some good friends who live a few doors away to see if they had any chocolate biscuits. There's a shop only two minutes away, but if I went to the shop and bought the biscuits myself I'd have the extra guilt of having deliberately acquired the offending items on top of the crime of eating them. If I just 'borrow' some from my pals then it's not that big a deal. I don't have to face the fact that I wanted them enough to go out and buy them. And anyway, crucially, if I went and bought them then there'd be the rest of the packet in the house and I can't have that here, because I'd just eat it. Whereas if I get a few from someone else, then I hold no responsibility for them, nor am I held to ransom by the packet. A proper fat person buys and eats a whole packet of biscuits. And although I think of myself as fat, I'm not fat enough in my head to go out and buy biscuits, just like that.

Tellingly, I tend not to make friends with other over-indulgers – evidently there's only room in my life for one hand in the cookie jar, as it were. I should confess that I don't like sharing. It makes me panic. My excuse for that would be that there was no sharing in my family (families, presumably, being where others learn the art of sharing). In my family we were pitched against each other for everything and in my case, particularly, for the right to eat, so it's hardly any wonder that sharing is problematic for me. I'm working on it, though. I'm drawn to people who are in control and able to do things in moderation. That way they can care for me. And that's part of the appeal of obliteration, too: finding someone who'll help you get there – a partner in crime but a guiltless one, someone who'll happily have a meal or a drink with you but isn't quite as reckless as you are. Really, I guess, someone who'll make sure everything doesn't completely unravel when you get obliterated, some-one who'll keep the world turning while you wobble out. As a mum does, I suppose, the ideal mum.

Everyone's got an opinion

Being fat is like having an unruly dog or a badly behaved child in public. There it is, for everyone to see, running amok, flamboyantly parading its bad upbringing, showing the world what a crap job you've done of disciplining it. Why, it's positively inviting others to have an opinion about how it's dealt with. Being fat makes you public property.

As anyone who's been anything from noticeably over-weight to morbidly obese for any length of time will know, it's tantamount to wearing a badge which says, 'Feel free to say what you think about what I'm eating or the way I look, because just by being fat I've given you licence to do so.' It's as if you've asked for it. Over the years, I have found that, without invitation or even an appropriate conversational opening, people have talked to me about my weight as if it were their right. The assumption also seems to be that I'm less sensitive to personal comments, since by being fat one is also usually considered to be 'jolly'. (And if not actually jolly, then certainly prepared to talk about the 'problem', since the person offering their opinion often seems to think they are being solicitous – a good friend – by bringing it to your attention.)

My experience involves a variety of people, some of whom, one would think, should have known better, and also a few . . . well, wankers. When I was 21, I went to Newcastle Playhouse to do a season in a repertory of plays. I was to play three parts in three different plays. During rehearsals the director (a woman) and the choreographer of the musical we were putting on openly discussed my weight, and the need for me to lose some. I never once objected. I thought they were right – I did need to lose weight, as I saw it, and ought to get on with doing so. I never questioned their position, never once thought, Shouldn't you have picked someone thinner, if that's what you wanted, when I auditioned for this season? The possibility of expressing such an idea (never mind having it in the first place) was light years away for me at that time. I felt very lucky to have the job and, moreover, lucky that they'd given it to me even though I was fat.

One day during rehearsals, I was standing in the unlit wings waiting to go on stage when the lead guy, a handsome, square-jawed, Gillette-man type, sidled up to me and whispered saucily in my ear, 'Hey, is it true that bigger girls need more sex?' I felt sick. Sure, I wanted him to fancy me; he was the lead man, and he was gorgeous. But it was sickening to be approached like that, as a 'big' girl who was clearly hungry all the time for everything, including sex. I wish I'd had the poise to reply, 'More sex than what?' But I didn't. I was embarrassed and tongue-tied, not least because I was absolutely sure that he wouldn't have made that sort of graceless overture to a thin girl. No, thin girls would require more elegance, more courting, more style; they're not 'asking for it' by being large, and therefore more sexually rapacious. I apparently warranted this comment simply by being overweight.

In my leaner years (professionally, not weightwise, natch), I used to do some secretarial work for a female local government councillor. She was bright, attractive, and independent. She was divorced and in no great hurry to find another man, being far too busy with politics and local causes. One day we were having lunch together in her kitchen. She picked up the tub of hummus we were eating and read the label. 'My God!' she cried, dropping the tub as if it had caught fire. 'Hummus has more fat than cheese!'

'Yeah, everyone knows that!' I said as I munched away merrily on my hummus-laden carrot stick. 'Hummus is really fattening.'

'But *you* eat it,' she said, without pausing for thought. She couldn't fathom how an overweight person would knowingly eat something 'fattening'. How did she think I'd got fat in the first place, I wondered?

I have a friend who's got an extremely high-profile job in journalism. He is highly intelligent. That is, professionally. There are usually gaps of several months between our meetings, and the last time we met I realised he'd lost a couple of stone and complimented him on how good he looked. 'Thanks!', he said. 'You should try this diet. It's really easy to do!' Leaving aside the fact that I hadn't asked him how I too could lose weight, he was, of course, conveniently forgetting that he has a wife at home to prepare and monitor his meals, and a PA to get his lunch and arrange his dinner engagements. In other words, someone else wrangles food and, indeed, temptation for him.

My mother, unsurprisingly I guess, was a great one for pointing out the bleeding obvious to people. The 50-year-old daughter of some very old friends of hers, a woman hereafter to be known as B, dutifully visited my mother regularly after her own parents had died. B is good company, well read, and pursues a very wide range of interests. B is also extremely big. She graduated from Oxford with a double first and now has a high-powered job in the Civil Service. She has, as far as one can tell, never had a relationship, and spends most of her free time with gay men with whom she also holidays. There are clearly some issues; but since she's not asking for help, whether or not she deals with them is her call, I'd say. After all, it's not as if she's stupid.

One day, however, after one of her visits, Mum asked me if she should tell B how 'very fat' she was.

'What, because she won't already know?' I asked sarcastically. 'It'll have escaped her attention and all she needs is a helpful little pointer from you? She's going to be *so* relieved when you tell her.'

Naturally, my mother ignored this. 'But she's *enormously* overweight. It's *so* bad for her health. She must do something about it.' And Mum won't have been the first person who wanted to let B know how fat she was. From Mum's perspective B's size was positively 'inviting' her to say something. At the same time, she had several friends who drank a great deal, yet she never suggested alerting them to the 'problem' of their alcoholism. It's as if 'fat' offends more than other physically manifested troubles.

Only a few days before she died, in her hospital bed, knowing how ill she was, Mum still couldn't help herself remarking on the sandwich I'd brought in for lunch. And only the other day, my not-fat-nor-ever-has-been sister told me not to eat the crackling off the pork joint.

A few years ago in America, a woman whose hugely overweight teenage daughter eventually died of organ failure was prosecuted for 'allowing' her child to eat so much it killed her. Her defence lawyer successfully argued for her acquittal on the grounds that no one is ever prosecuted for the many anorexia-related deaths that occur every year, since being too thin isn't seen as being as heinous as being too fat. Notwithstanding that it is a mental illness, the self-imposed deprivation central to anorexia confers an element of martyrdom, whereas there's nothing self-sacrificial, i.e. 'worthy', about self-imposed overindulgence.

Society admires painfully thin celebrities while it points an accusing finger at the obese ones. When the singer Beth Ditto wore a very tight Lycra dress on stage, a tabloid newspaper wrote, 'A fearless Beth Ditto, 28, squeezed herself into the tight-fitting Lycra frock, testing its limits almost to the point of destruction ... But even for Ditto – whose love of tight clothing appears to have no boundaries – this was a look too far, as the frock failed to flatter her 15st figure.' This was in a newspaper whose huge readership mainly consists of women, yet there were no complaints about the piece's message: fat girls shouldn't wear revealing dresses. At least it seems that a sort of backlash (although it's hardly huge) is slowly beginning, with a number of blogs started by 'bigger' girls who are interested in fashion and looking for a way of expressing their rage at how marginalised they are.

There was an ad for Maltesers on TV in the Seventies which my friends and I all used to take off at school. It depicted a casual group – one guy and two girls – sitting in their swimsuits at a table next to a public swimming pool. Another girl approached the group, eating a bag of Maltesers. One of the seated girls cried out 'Chocolate?!', in a tone clearly intended to suggest a subtext of 'You fat cow, not caring about your weight and, worse, in a swimsuit.' The guilty chocolate-eater smilingly replied, 'No, Maltesers!' Now, as I'm sure you're aware, a key ingredient of Maltesers is, in fact, chocolate, but the Malteser-eater's casual tone suggested everyone could relax – no need for worry! She wasn't a porker, unaware of the hidden pitfalls of eating chocolate, for this wasn't fattening chocolate like some (fat) girls eat; these were Maltesers, 'the sweet with the less fattening centre', as the catchphrase went back then, and therefore *wholly* different from the fattening chocolate a girl not taking care of herself might eat!

Even back then, when, with every fibre of my being, I truly believed I had to be thinner to be everything I yearned to be – better, worthier, prettier, everything-ier – my friends and I thought that ad was funny. It was the way the word 'Chocolate?!' was used to convey shock and disgust, and the relief expressed upon discovering that Maltesers were, in fact, a *less fattening* chocolate.

The message that you mustn't get fat is reinforced by the way much of the media discuss women even today.

These publications openly debate celebrities' weight, whether too fat or too thin, and, exclusively in relation to women, their 'imperfections'. Every edition of every one of these magazines will include sections entitled 'Cellulite watch', 'Bony knees', or 'Too fat for a bikini?' Each one of them invites the reader to judge the featured celebrity unfavourably. The message is pernicious: women need to look a very specific and impossible-to-achieve way in order to avoid being criticised and in some cases written off. With a constant onslaught of advertising, shows featuring 'perfect' girls and the glut of popular magazines on sale, girls and women are being fed a strong message: that the way we look matters more than anything else we have to offer.

You might think these magazines are a bit of a laugh – harmless fun – and that you don't take these ritualistic public outings of women's 'fat bits' seriously. That may very well be so, but the fact is that poor body image, low self-esteem, and eating disorders are very much on the rise, particularly in teenage girls. There has been a sharp increase in the number of young girls being admitted to hospital in England for anorexia. Statistics released in response to a parliamentary question show an 80 per cent rise in sufferers aged 16 or under between 2006 and 2007. Shockingly, there was also a 207 per cent rise in hospitalisations for 12-year-olds with eating disorders.

Overall, the message is clear. If you don't want to draw unwelcome attention to yourself, then don't be fat. Oh yes, and don't eat chocolate – least of all in a swimsuit.

Passive-aggressive pudding

Popular comedy would have us believe that, in general, mothers of boys take an instant dislike to their darling sons' girlfriends. I've had plenty of boyfriends and little experience of that myth. In fact, I've often ended up liking my boyfriends' mothers more than the boyfriends. However, some mothers do have 'em, or rather some of 'em do have some mothers, and there are those who won't like you no matter how wonderful you may or may not be.

I went out with one guy who had an unusually intense relationship with his mother and, even before we were introduced, it was clear she did not like 'sharing' him. He was sweet and great in many ways but turned out to be pathologically immature, so a proper relationship really wasn't possible. For example, he'd been away working abroad for weeks and when he got back he wanted to watch *Dumb and Dumber* rather than have welcome-home sex – and it was a DVD, so, you know, he could have watched it later. Even organising a cinema date a week in advance made him panic that it might lead to marriage. (I know I don't come off too well here, either, but my thinking, at the time, was that you usually have to go in for some 'model modifications', don't you?)

After we had been seeing each other for a few months, he announced that his mother would like to meet me. I should have spotted the fatal error immediately. He didn't say, 'I'd like you to meet my mother' but, much more tellingly and frankly worryingly, 'My mother wants to meet you.' He was an only son and, I got the impression, the apple of her eye. But at the time, I took the offer as an indication of greater commitment, and readily agreed. He called his mother right then and there and she suggested we come for lunch the following Sunday.

Just as they were ending the call I heard him say, 'I'll ask her.' He turned to me. 'Mum's asking if there's anything you don't like to eat.'

Call me over-sensitive, but I instantly suspected it was a trap. Why would she ask a question like that unless she was planning on serving up monkey brains? What motive could she possibly have for asking that, other than to flush me out as an ungrateful, picky princess who makes unreasonable demands of all her hostesses before she's even set foot inside their front door?

Not wanting to be caught out, I simply shrugged my shoulders nonchalantly and made an 'Everything's fine' face. Anyway, I couldn't think of anything I didn't like enough to have it relayed to my boyfriend's mother, apart from blancmange and tripe. In that moment I reasoned that these two not-generally-much-seen items weren't very likely to appear together, on the same menu, at my boyfriend's mother's house on a Sunday lunchtime.

'Nothing, she says anything's fine,' the boyfriend said to his mother happily. Clearly, Mummy Dearest wasn't having that. 'Oh, OK,' he said, and turned to me again. 'Mum says you should just say, she won't mind, she says she'd rather know.' It was definitely a trap, I was sure of it. But in the interest of good relations I elected to take her at her word and be honest.

'Well, I don't really like any eggy, custardy dishes.' (I loathe trifle, crème brûlée, blancmange – I can't stand anything that moves in my mouth.)

The boyfriend passed on the information, which was, apparently, met with good humour and that was the end of it. 'Mum's a fantastic cook – it should be a great meal,' he said, replacing the receiver.

The following Sunday, we met up to go to his mother's. I'd brought a nice bunch of flowers and so had he. His flowers were nicer than mine. Never mind, I felt sure she'd be pleased to get not one but two bunches of flowers. At first Mummy Dearest was rather formal, a bit frosty even. It didn't help that she looked at my flowers as if they'd been bought at the traffic lights, while greeting his bunch as if he'd fashioned each individual flower himself from origami. I didn't feel very at ease and she was certainly making no effort to alter that.

For all that turned out to be not right about this boyfriend in terms of a relationship with me, he was a very bouncy, friendly guy, so I was surprised by his mother's *froideur*. She was originally from Paris, so I decided that was probably why she was being a bit snooty and comforted myself with the knowledge that she was, apparently, a really good cook. And her being French only added to the belief. After a bit of awkward chitchat she invited us to sit down to the lunch.

The first course was a lovely joint of beef with vegetables and potatoes dauphinoise, and all was well. The conversation was a little stilted, not greatly helped by the boyfriend and his mother lapsing into very fast, colloquial French (it has to be said, instigated by her). She didn't know that, in fact, I can speak a little French, but I couldn't keep up with this. I think the boyfriend was a bit embarrassed by his mother's obvious efforts to exclude me, but I couldn't be sure and he obviously wanted to keep her onside.

'*Alors, maintenant, la pièce de résistance, le dessert,*' Madame de Pompidou announced, scraping back her chair and gathering herself to her full, stiff-backed height. You'd have thought she was about to produce a soufflé timed to within an inch of its life, she was so grave and ceremonial about it. I started getting quite excited: it must be something great, surely, since she'd hardly be making such a song and dance about something simple like an apple pie, would she? I love most puddings anyway and was salivating at the prospect of something absolutely wonderful.

'*Oeufs à la neige!*' she pronounced solemnly, lowering a huge cut-crystal punch bowl on to the table as carefully and slowly as if she were producing the baby Jesus. The bowl was filled to the brim with a creamy viscous liquid that looked worryingly like breast milk. There were bits floating in it and they looked distinctly egg-shaped. The 'breast milk' swayed gently, lapping the sides of the bowl as it settled to a glassy calm. Suddenly, I remembered that *oeuf* was French for egg. They looked like bleached sheep's droppings. I thought I was going to heave.

'Can I serve you some, Arabella?' the boyfriend's mother asked with all the faux innocence she could muster. We both knew it was a test. She'd deliberately made a pudding containing only the very things she'd been told I hated. I decided then and there that she'd have cooked whatever she'd been told I didn't like. It was a trap, just as I'd thought, and I'd played right into her hands – I'd given her the eggs with which to lay it! I knew she'd like me more if I ate it. But even though at that stage I was still keen on her son, I did not have it in me to clear this hurdle. It was a pistols-at-dawn standoff, except it was poached egg whites at about 2 p.m. on a rainy Sunday afternoon. It was true, she'd caught me out: I didn't like her son enough to eat a poached egg white floating in breast milk. I didn't like *anyone* enough to eat it.

I looked at her, willing her to read my thoughts: I know you know that I know you made that pudding with the specific intention of showing me up as ill mannered and at the same time demonstrating how little I deserve your precious son. It turns out, I'm not so good at telepathy because she said nothing but smiled sweetly, a large serving spoon poised over the *oeufs*. I panicked. I didn't want to insult her cooking, but I *really* didn't want to eat it. I couldn't.

And then it came to me, a brainwave, something she'd surely admire more than eating a pudding she already knew

I hated just to be polite. 'Sorry, no, it looks absolutely delicious!' I said, 'but I'm on a diet.'

Hah! I felt in my bones that she'd want her son's girl-friend to have a more conventionally attractive figure than mine. I could just sense that she hadn't liked my roundness from the moment she'd seen me walk through the door. Now the dilemma was hers: should she urge me to break my 'diet' with this delicious pudding, and thereby suggest that my figure was fine with her? I was sure she was torn between trying to torture me with her revolting concoction and wanting me to be thinner.

However, she was clearly made of sterner stuff. 'It's a great French delicacy!' she persisted.

'And it is very tempting,' I lied, 'but I really need to lose some weight, so, you know . . .'

She'd meticulously planned a win-win situation – if I ate the pudding, I proved that I sought her approval of me enough to eat something she knew I didn't like. However, by eating it I would also show that I didn't care enough about her son to take care of my figure for him. On the other hand, if I rejected the pudding it showed that I cared more about my own likes and dislikes than about her son and was therefore, via a different route, revealing myself to be not good enough for him.

But, with this brilliant counter strike, I'd won. I knew I had. I could feel it. Victory was mine. And sweet enough to make up for the pudding I hadn't had. My 'diet' had rescued me from her cunning plan.

On the way home, the boyfriend looked sulky. 'You might at least have tried Mum's pudding. It's her speciality.

You hurt her feelings. She'd made it specially for you.' I looked at him, silently imploring him to remember. He returned my look with that of a wounded puppy and I realised he'd forgotten. He'd genuinely forgotten that the dreaded pudding was made of the very things I'd been so insistently urged to confess I didn't like. I decided not to fight it.

'Yeah, well, it looked very fattening and I am on a diet. I'd just decided.'

The boyfriend smiled warmly at me. 'Good, I'm glad to hear it,' he replied, patting me on the leg.

So then I hated him *and* his mother.

Flying spaghetti

Look, I know I can be annoying. Of course I can. I'm very opinionated, I talk a lot, possibly even all the time, often speak before I've thought through what I'm going to say ('simply for the pleasure of hearing your own voice', my dad used to say), and, in an argument, I can be unreasonably reluctant to back down. I know my faults. (OK, possibly not all my faults; if I did I probably wouldn't see the point of getting up in the morning.) Let us say that I'm aware that I can be annoying – but then, can't everyone?

If, however, you are brought up believing that *everything* you do is annoying, then it follows that you'll believe everything is your fault. On a bigger scale, and in my experience, women blame themselves when things go wrong much more readily than men. And if that is your default mode, then trying to fashion new, healthier, more rational reactions takes time and a great deal of presence of mind – and, hey, maybe even some support from your friends and family.

Of my slightly-too-many-equal-in-awfulness-to-be-all-their-fault bad boyfriends, number two was an Italian. Following a few happy months of employment in a regional theatre, I rewarded myself (yes, I'm afraid actors only work for a few weeks before they feel entitled to a 'break') with a trip to Italy to visit my friend Michele, whom I'd met hitch-hiking years earlier. Michele is an electrician and lighting designer, and lives in the country in a tiny house next to a church about 12 miles outside Florence. There, one night, I met one of his colleagues, a handsome man with kind eyes called Gilberto.

I was 32, and at a crossroads: was my life really going to be an on-off limp between occasional not-very-exciting acting jobs and temping as a secretary? Surely this wasn't *it*? With Gilberto was his seven-year-old son, Niccolo, with whom I hit it off instantly. He was bouncy, friendly, and chatty and, exhausted from his day at school, he curled up next to me on the sofa within ten minutes of meeting me. I was enchanted. As Niccolo fell asleep in my lap his father and I got talking, had a few drinks and ate some nice food, and a few days later we got together. Gilberto was divorced and had his son with him for half of each week. This was just the opening I'd been subconsciously looking for, and, more than willingly, I fell into becoming a step-mother to Niccolo. Over the next 18 months I commuted between Italy and England, staying in London only to earn a bit of money before rushing back to Italy to be with my new 'family'.

Gilberto was a sensational cook, and for a while he was madly in love with me. I basked in the warm sunshine of his fevered attention and developed a close, loving relationship with Niccolo. And, of course, adding to the appeal of my life in Italy was the fact that there I was no longer a slightly-too-fat, out-of-work actress in London: I was spending more than half my time in a beautiful hot country where I had a proper role – caring for a child.

Had I not adored Niccolo, I'd like to think I'd have left the relationship with his dad when it started to go bad. Actually, that's not true – I'm saying that as if I've ever been the sort of woman who walked away from relationships that weren't 'good' for her, like the heroine of an uplifting and charming movie. The reality is that I'd probably have stayed on indefinitely if Gilberto hadn't chucked me in the end. I've always stayed until the bitter end, even after I've stopped wanting to be with them. I can't do chucking – I'm too worried that I might change my mind later, only to find the option's no longer there. It's a kind of hoarding, another version of ensuring your supply. So worried was I that, not entitled, as I felt, to choice, I'd end up with nothing, I'd 'keep' boyfriends I no longer wanted just to have something safe.

So there I was, slightly surprised to find myself a full-time stepmother and housewife, kidding myself all the while that it was meaningful when really it was a fantasy, an escape from real life in the UK. Eventually, Gilberto's passion began to wane but I clung on, desperate not to have to go back to London and my old life again.

One night, towards the end of the relationship, we'd invited my mother and her old friend Hazel over to dinner. Mum and Hazel had been students together in Italy in the early Fifties and Hazel had married an Italian, settling in

Florence, where Mum often visited her. Naturally, since he was such a good cook, Gilberto was making that night's meal, but he'd asked me to do the shopping while he was at work. Now, I spoke Italian fairly fluently, but I'm not a good cook, and nor do I care about the shape, size, and texture of things, the science of it all. On Gilberto's shopping list was the item 'spaghetti' and, uninitiated as I was in the finer details of his menu for the night, spaghetti was what I bought.

When Mum and Hazel arrived, there was still no sign of Gilberto, and I couldn't help thinking he was making a point, showing me how little he cared about being polite. Eventually he sailed in, waved at our guests in semi-but-clearly-not-genuine apology, and immediately embarked on a display of flamboyant cooking. There ensued an impressive whirlwind of chopping and banging of pots and pans, loudly peppered with demands to be brought this and that. (In my experience, most men cook in a similar show-off style – 'Hey, look at me, I'm cooking!' – just like little boys on swings: 'Hey, Mum, look at me, see how high I'm going, it's really exciting!' That's why so many 'great' professional cooks are men; it's just another way of waving their willies around, shouting, 'Hey, get a load of this! I'm brilliant!' Maybe it's because, unfettered as they are by the tyranny of believing they need to be thin to be sexy (unlike women), they're not plagued by concerns that the ingredients will make them fat – they are physiologically less likely to put on weight, for starters. When dreaming up dishes, they are able to let their warrior side loose and they can approach cooking with nothing but pure brio.)

Mum, Hazel, and I are chatting and drinking wine at the table while Gilberto chargrills aubergines and courgettes. He's chopping fresh parsley with a flourish, he's got some cream on to simmer, the water's on the boil, it's all go. All that's left to do is the spaghetti. I point to the cupboard where I've dutifully put away all the dry goods from his list and continue the conversation with our guests.

Suddenly Gilberto, brandishing the packet of spaghetti as if it were a truncheon, yells at me, 'What the *fuck* is this?'

We all fall silent. 'Spaghetti,' I say. Our guests seem satisfied with the answer, for, after all, that is what it appears to be.

But that's not right. Gilberto hurls the bag of spaghetti across the room. It flies in an arc like a falling star. He's shouting. 'For fuck's sake, it's number 12, not number 10!'

Now, I'd spent a lot of time in Italy, and a great deal of that with my friend Michele, who is also a sensational cook. Nevertheless, I had absolutely no idea what Gilberto was talking about. Evidently, my blank expression made my ignorance clear.

'This is *spaghettini*, not spaghetti. I can't make this dish with spaghettini! Can't you do *anything* properly? Not even the shopping?'

I waited for the laugh that was surely coming any minute now. There wasn't one. He wasn't joking. Apparently, I had failed to compare the word on his list with the word on the bag of pasta for a forensic match, as any conscientious housewife should. I looked to our guests for support. Hazel was staring intently into her wineglass. My mother, meanwhile, was looking at me, eyebrows raised, with an expectant expression. I decided not to say anything in my defence, because clearly there wasn't one.

However, we still had to have supper. Naturally, Gilberto couldn't climb down from his high horse to walk across the room and pick up the hurled spaghetti. He couldn't make do; a man of passion does not 'make do' with the only spaghetti available, wrong circumference notwithstanding. So, like a giant dog turd on the pavement, the bag of spaghetti remained on the floor where it had landed. It was not mentioned again. Since the pasta couldn't be used we ate bread (I don't recall what size it was) with the sauce, and very good it was, too.

Later, as I saw Mum and Hazel to their car, I whispered conspiratorially, looking for support and hoping to make up for the scene they'd had to endure, 'Sorry about that pathetic display. Bloody hell, it was only spaghetti . . .'

My mother shook her head despondently, as if I'd utterly missed the point. 'No, darling, food is very important to the Italians and you *did* buy the wrong size spaghetti.'

Outing my bum

Just as, in my youth (well, really, always), I believed that I couldn't expect to attract the interest of cool boys because I lacked the correct qualifications (i.e. being thin and pretty), I spent my entire acting career knowing that real success would elude me for as long as I failed to look like Greta Scacchi, to pick at random one of my aforementioned more conventionally attractive contemporaries.

Actually, she's not a random choice at all. I probably ought to confess that I have a 'thing' about her, or did, anyway. I'm over it now – really I am, *honestly*. We met once; actually, we didn't really meet as such. I happened to be with a producer she knew at the theatre one night, and they chatted while I stood by, feeling like an industrial-sized bag of potatoes. She was everything I wanted to be: slim, beautiful, and, even though it was a first night, casually dressed, looking completely, effortlessly ravishing in a pair of faded jeans and a white shirt. She was fresh from her success in the movie *White Mischief* and very much in demand. I was very much . . . not.

But it wasn't jealousy of her fame or looks that sparked my ire. My 'thing' about her materialised when the producer asked what project she was now busy with. 'Actually, it's a nightmare,' she sighed wearily. 'It's just scripts, scripts, scripts . . . I simply don't have the time to read everything I'm offered!' The image of her wading through a trough of scripts grated on me. From my stunningly script-and-offer-free perspective at the time it didn't seem as though that would be a nightmare at all.

It seemed a little grand to be complaining about how much work she had, as if it were a burden – particularly in a profession notorious for massive unemployment. Who knows, though? Perhaps there's every chance that, had I been equally in demand, my disgruntlement at the mountain of 'chores' she was facing would never have seen the light of day.

Silly or not (and even leaving Ms Scacchi aside), the fact remains that the size of my arse ruled my life. And, of course, added to the list were my saggy boobs, fat stomach, rampant cellulite, and the rest. But these, erm, 'features' could be hidden from view with some clever dressing. The bum, however, simply could not be tamed. No control pants, no tight skirt with inner panels, no size-too-small-squishing-it-all-in trousers were capable of masking the fact that it was there, and it was big.

Since I believed that its bigness was *the* principal obstacle that lay between me and success, I invented some clever strategies for dealing with auditions. I am able to report, hand on heart, that my favoured option was a cleverly, and heavily rehearsed, handbag manoeuvre. I exited many, many audition rooms ensuring that the handbag, chosen specifically for its size, swung around my shoulder as I turned towards the door and came to rest over my arse, thereby masking its gigantic proportions. I was absolutely sure, assuming the audition had otherwise gone well, that catching sight of my huge arse would instantly scupper my chances by causing my prospective employers to change their minds about me (and, as I saw it, rightly so).

And don't imagine for one moment that I executed this necessary (so I believed) tactic with any lightness of spirit. I didn't do this to be funny. I didn't think it *was* funny. It was deadly serious. The size of my bum embodied all that I felt was wrong with me. If anyone saw it, my cover would be blown, because they'd instantly realise exactly why I ought not to be allowed to join their club.

Imagine my surprise, then, when my big arse turned out to be the very thing that led to eventual success. I struggle to believe that the bum that had dominated my every waking moment, that I had worked so hard to hide, ended up opening the door for me. I had spent the first ten years of my career doing everything on earth (except, of course, losing any real weight) on the run from my bum and its perceived sabotaging of my career. And then, in a moment of madness, I make a joke about it in front of other people and everything changes.

Until then I'd had various spurts of success – a theatre job here, a telly job there – but there'd been no continuity, no sense of development. Some of these jobs were quite good, high profile even, but I still hadn't had enough continuous employment or the kind of recognition that would validate my career as a performer. That didn't happen until the first series of *The Fast Show*, when Paul (Whitehouse) and Charlie (Higson) casually suggested I write someone who was *like me*.

'What do you mean, like me?' I asked innocently. I couldn't think what they meant.

'You know, always wondering if the most important thing about her is how fat she looks,' they replied, as one.

Mmm. Clearly, they'd talked about my obsessions behind my back (behind my bum, even). But, amazingly, I didn't recognise the woman they were describing. That's not how I saw myself. I didn't see my 'problems' with any kind of levity. I saw them as real, permanent impediments, not something that I or others might joke about. Luckily for me, though, I didn't storm out of the room in indignant hurt that they were treating my problems with such casual disregard. I started thinking that they might be right: there might be comic mileage in a character who, no matter where she found herself (a court of law, giving birth, taking the sacrament, anywhere, everywhere), would wonder if the way she looked was pivotal to the proceedings. And eventually, I decided on a catchphrase that captured all her anxieties: 'Does my bum look big in this?'

I can't pretend that this was an epiphany. By writing that catchphrase, I wasn't actively deciding to 'out' *it*, as it were. This wasn't the moment when I finally dropped the handbag manoeuvre and admitted I had a fat arse. It just seemed like the best catchphrase for this character (by now called Insecure Woman). And it wasn't until I started writing the various sketches in which I played different types of 'everywoman' – a judge, a doctor, a parking warden, and so on – that I realised that my bum, my own actual real-life bum, in all its enormous glory, would be the focus of attention for the TV-watching nation. By accident, as it were, I was now positively inviting people to scrutinise the very thing I'd spent my entire adult life hiding.

Fortunately, Insecure Woman and her catchphrase took off. The TV-watching nation, it turned out, could relate to her arse and her worries. So, after the show, I wrote a book using the catchphrase as its title. And by the time the publisher wanted ideas for the book's cover, I had realised (about bloody time, you might say) that there was just no getting away from the bum. So, again to my surprise, I decided to appear naked on the cover. I couldn't think of any other way to convey the utter vulnerability of a woman who feels insecure about her own body. And the book sold incredibly well – again, to my amazement, because as I was writing it I'd spent the whole time asking myself if there was really likely to be anyone else in the world as bonkers as I was about my body and food.

You'd think that, after all that validation, I'd have felt liberated – out and proud. You'd be wrong. I was delighted and gratified that the character in the show and the book did so well, but none of that meant that I suddenly learnt to love my bum. That would have been ridiculous. Sure, the bum had paid for itself; but it hadn't turned into something I could be proud of. Only the loss of 20 pounds and a complete redesign could have made that happen.

However, the success I'd found by laying out my

insecurities for all to see did eventually change the way I saw myself in the wider world. And although it's only too apparent that women are still a long way from being free of the burden of being judged above all else for the way they look, I, for one, now believe that I have something to offer even though I'm not thin.

It took me a long time to let go of my trusty neuroses. After all, they'd been my 'thing' for a very long time. They'd been the reasons I'd been able to hold up to explain all that was wrong with my life. For all those years, I hadn't had to look any further than 'I'm fat, and fat people don't get what thin people get'. Although I still think (and there's a lot of evidence to support this thinking) that there are a great many prejudices attached to being fat, I don't think now that my own particular rotund shape was the only block to my chances of realising my potential. I'd become so accustomed to the idea that fatness was the *one* thing wrong with me that I didn't have to look at anything else. That was it: everything bad came from being fat, and everything good would come if I weren't. So I was told. Naturally enough then, the professional success I eventually achieved didn't immediately cancel out this equation, because by the equation's own unforgiving terms it was my success that didn't add up. How on earth could I be successful while I was still fat?

Eventually, I realised that I'd unearthed what I was good at by exposing my fears and what I really was. By letting my belt out a few notches, figuratively speaking, I could stop holding my stomach in, breathe out, and focus on bigger and better things.

The paparazzi were doing a full back shot of me in a swimsuit and I thought, 'Oh my God, I have to be so brave.' See, every woman hates herself from behind.

Cindy Crawford

Don't eat pudding if you want to get a job (or a boyfriend)

While writing this book I've naturally started thinking (even more than I did already) about why and how I eat, and especially why and how I overeat, on the occasions when I do. And I've realised something I'd never stopped to think about before: that I wouldn't eat pudding in front of someone I either fancied or hoped would employ me.

I wanted to know whether I was unique in this deceit. (Well, it is a form of deceit, isn't it? If I'm the sort of person who does eat pudding, potential suitors or employers might as well know that from the off.) So I asked nine of my girl-friends, whose body shapes range from extremely thin to well covered, if they'd eat pudding on a first date or at a business lunch. Every single one of them said 'No'. And most then added, 'But I don't know why.'

So it turns out that, as I'd suspected, women censor their eating instinctively. We automatically think we will be less attractive, both sexually and professionally, if we're seen to be gluttonous. I asked a similar number of male friends the same question. Every single one of them, without pausing for thought, looked at me as if I were mad and said, 'Why wouldn't I?' Boys are not brought up to make a connection between their physical appeal and the relative likelihood of getting a partner or a job. Girls are.

And it's not just me and my friends who think this: there's actual proof. Imagine my delight when, hoping to back up the findings of my amateur 'pudding poll', I came across a scientific research paper entitled 'What You Eat Depends on Your Sex and Eating Companions'. Result! As you might suspect, all of us, men and women, are likely to eat more when we eat in company than we do alone. Eating is a social event, so it stands to reason that we eat more with others than we do if we're alone. However, 'women, but not men, eat significantly less when with opposite-sex strangers.' The report goes on to state that 'women are deemed more attractive' and (wait for it) 'more feminine when portrayed as eating fewer calories'. And finally, get this: 'women's choice of food is significantly influenced by whether eating companions were only other women or both sexes'. In other words, they ate what they wanted if they were eating with girlfriends, but 'watched' what they ate if eating with men.

So the old joke is true! Q: 'What would the world be without men?' A: 'Full of fat, happy women.' (And, in case you didn't already know it, there's this at the end of the research report: 'Social status and wealth affect men's romantic appeal to women more than physical attractiveness.' Thank heavens someone's finally cleared up the mystery of how old, bald, rich guys get gorgeous young girls . . .)

I'm not saying it's men's fault we can't seem to get comfortable with eating pudding in front of them – nor that it's their fault that overweight women are unhappy with themselves. Actually, judging by the reaction that old joke gets, it's more our fault than theirs. Non-slim girls and women are by a wide margin the vast majority in the developed world, yet we seem happy, or at least willing, to participate in the belief that we can and should reduce our size to something we're extremely unlikely ever to be able to achieve. To paraphrase Betty Friedan, the mother of the feminist movement, 'women are being duped into believing being thin is their natural destiny'.

And, hey, it's not just the boyfriend you won't get if you eat the cake: it's the job or the promotion as well! Yup, I'm sorry to have to tell you that there's proper research (see, not just me whingeing) to back this up. A study which collated data from 29 separate research papers found that, while 61 per cent of top male bosses were overweight, the same was true of just 22 per cent of women in similar jobs. The research revealed that overweight workers were routinely stereotyped as 'possessing negative personality traits and as emotionally impaired. They were considered to be lazy, out of control and dirty ... overweight women elicited the most negative reactions.' 93 per cent of human resources professionals said they would give a job to the thinner person out of two equally able candidates. And how's this for proof, if proof were needed, that it's definitely much worse for women: 'being overweight harms only females ... there is a tendency to hold women to harsher weight standards'. Gosh, really?

Here's another joke. It's awful but in many ways true. Q: 'What's the only thing men and women have in common?' A: 'They all hate women.' And surely, self-hatred must have something to do with why we all buy into the tyranny of 'thin is good, fat is bad'. Oh, but it's such an endlessly tough tug-of-war between the allure of a new you and the prospect of facing the reality that this is who you are and that's OK. Who wants 'OK' when you could have *brilliant*?! 'Thin' as the ultimate state of being is shoved down our throats every minute of every day. (Don't worry, it's calorie-free.)

Dieting is marketed as easy, achievable, and, wow, even fun! But we ought, really, to see dieting for what it really is: a con. The appeal of a new 'miracle' diet is just like the thrill you get from flicking through a lifestyle magazine. It's saying to you, 'Hey, you know what? You can have a brand-new you by simply acquiring these things. No effort, no sweat, no heartache – just purchase.' We're all guilty of being sucked in, of thinking, Yes! If I get all those pink boxfiles, I will *instantly* have a pink boxfile kind of life! There'll be no stained toilet bowls, no grumpy bosses or partners, no last-minute laddered tights – it'll all be fresh, new, and lovely! We have exactly the same feelings when we embark on a new diet. 'I can do it! This time I'm going to get myself a new body!' And when I do I'll get that job, boyfriend, promotion – the perfect life.

Every single diet on the market puts forward the notion that this is the one that will be your friend – the one who knows you, who can help you lose weight, an answer to all your problems, finally, and you can rely on it 100 per cent.

We're all looking for the oracle, whatever form it takes – anything, something, that'll take responsibility for all the troubling unanswerables in life. We all dream of a Dumbledore or a fairy godmother – a mythical, wise parent who'll lay to rest all our anxieties, and just *know* stuff. Diets offer that: the answer, the lure, the notion, the possibility that you actually aren't the 'you' who overeats sometimes, or puts on weight more easily than other people despite not eating very much. They beckon you in, offering an escape into another world where another, better 'you' awaits – and all you have to do to get there is to buy this diet book/pill/regime/exercise plan, etc. It all amounts to a business worth between 40 and 100 billion dollars a year – yes, a *year*. Now, the diet industry wouldn't be making that much money if there was one single diet that worked, would it? We'd all use that one, and that'd be the end of the multi-billion-dollar industry.

Having said all that, I am deeply ashamed to admit that all these negative reactions to 'fat women' sum up everything I once felt about Mum's size. Mum actually wasn't overweight at all. She was big boned and perhaps carried more weight than she had as a young woman. But, crucially I guess, in terms of how I saw her, she *thought* she was fat, and what's more she didn't like herself. She was a tall woman, with broad shoulders, long legs, and what they used to call a 'good bust'. She was handsome, too – in a womanly way, rather than pretty like a girl. There are some photos of her looking incredibly glamorous but that's not, I'm afraid, how I saw her when I was a teenager, nor even more sadly how she ever saw herself. I saw her, and she referred to herself as such, too, as a discarded woman, deserving of contempt for 'allowing' herself to be cast off by a successful, thin, glamorous, and (importantly) now absent man. Dad, of course, took on immense appeal simply by not being the one left trying and failing to deal with stroppy teenagers, a run-down house, loneliness, confusion, and a marriage in tatters.

And I'm afraid I did think that she was 'lazy, dirty, out of control'. As it happens, by her own admission later in life she *was* guilty of being those things, but not because of anything to do with her weight. She cheerfully admitted to having no interest in cleanliness if there was a book to be read, and not caring if things (be they clothes, bodies, or baths) were dirty or food was off.

For all Mum's faults and the difficulties between the two of us, I see now that she found herself alone and confused and, like most women then and today, she blamed a lot of what had happened on how she had 'failed' to be more conventionally slim and attractive. If only she could have been the sort of woman who had enough self-discipline to stay trim, make nice dinners, and not needle her husband. If only she could have been less like herself. And I wanted her to be more conventional, too. I wanted her to look less chaotic and *be* less chaotic; I wanted her to look like other friends' mums and make ordinary suppers as they did. Her very slight overweightness, such as it was, became a symbol of everything that was wrong, scary, and out of control in our house. Fat equalled destruction and the loss of everything nice and precious.

Sexual eating

Eating in the presence of a person with whom you're also trying to maintain sexual allure is always tricky for those of us with any kind of eating 'issues'. In the beginning, you've just met and it's all a bit unreal, in a good way. Suddenly, you're both soaring above ordinary folk and their humdrum ways, drunk on that heady, initial stage of being in love and both pretending to be something you're not. Perhaps 'pretending' is too negative a word. You may not be actively pretending, but you're certainly caught up in that unique phase when you believe anything's possible – that brand-new-beautiful-day feeling. We are all at our very best during those intoxicating first few weeks (months, if we're lucky) when we're getting to know someone who thrills us and makes us, in return, feel all skippy, shiny, and capable of anything. Capable of having sex three times a day, capable of watching the crummiest of TV shows together without getting bored, capable of not getting irritated by being stuck in a traffic jam together, capable of not being furious if they turn up late, capable of liking their unlikeable friends, capable of drinking beer because they do ... Capable of enjoying anything at all, including the soon-to-be intolerable.

When newly in love, historically I have turned into a person who does all of the above, but who also doesn't eat too much, doesn't eat pudding, and even, sometimes, doesn't eat at all. At the beginning of a new relationship, when my partner and I have been having sex with that uniquely unfeasible-in-the-long-term frequency, I haven't eaten nearly as much as I inevitably would, it turned out, later on in the relationship. Later on, when the person I really am has finally shown her face; when I've settled back into being me, when (it has to be said) I'm not trying so hard any more, and perhaps even can't be bothered to keep putting in the energy required to sustain that 'new me'.

And since I did think (and still do a lot of the time) that I *ought* to be thinner, it naturally followed that I'd expect a partner to (at the very least) *suggest* I consider not eating something like an éclair. (As it happens I don't eat éclairs very often. They're not really my treat of choice. I'm using an éclair here as a symbol of something containing absolutely no hunger-sating properties.) After all, if *I* think I'm a little bit fat, then surely he ought to, too, no? Who wants to be in a club that wants you as a member?

That extraordinarily pretty girl I knew at school, who later became a model, once told me she never ate on a date because 'Men don't like to see girls eat. It's not attractive.' Even at 17, I knew it was a silly thing to say, but couldn't help also envying her commitment to (and therefore superior knowledge of) doing 'what boys like' – and especially her ability to use this as a motivation to resist eating.

However, as time went on, it eventually dawned on me, through trial and error, that my fluctuating weight made no difference to the number of men who did or did not find me attractive. Nor, more importantly, did it make any difference to the quality of the relationship and my tendency to gauge who I was accordingly. I eventually settled into the place I am now: someone who eats and drinks more than she ought to, according to government guidelines, and could certainly lose a few pounds, again using those guidelines, but doesn't have enough commitment to (or interest in) 'what boys like' to miss out on nice food and wine on that account, nor is in dogged pursuit of the superior quality of life apparently only available to thin people. And it was from this resigned-to-the-facts-of-life position that I managed to form a relationship with a man, now my husband, on whom I didn't do the 'éclair test'.

Having said that, don't imagine it means for one moment that I'm now completely at home with my body or eating habits. I'm light years away from that enviable – you might say mythical – state of mind. I'm also still illogically angry that boys can, it would seem, eat so much more than girls. It's not fair. It would be a mite fairer if men and women had equal prospects in life relative to their abilities, but they don't.

For example, when my husband, who is trim and physically fit, strolls into the kitchen and makes his way towards the fridge with what I can instantly tell is an 'Is there any bacon?' swagger, all I feel is rage. I can always tell when he's about to make himself a big breakfast. There's a particular 'I'm entitled' strut. And it always annoys me. It isn't logical. It isn't a seasoned reaction to the familiar (but nonetheless fabulously irritating) routine of him not washing up the frying pan afterwards, or splattering the kitchen ceiling with grease as he hurls the entire packet of bacon and three eggs into the pan. It's not even the two whole bagels or six slices of toast heaped with at least half a packet of butter to go with the fry-up that gets my goat. That's not what makes my blood boil. Watching him prepare that . . . is 'meal' a big enough word for all that food? . . . without screaming requires absolutely all the willpower I'm able to muster. It's just that he *can*.

I used to kid myself that it *was* the mess, the self-indulgence equal to that of a Roman emperor, the swaggering display of entitlement to a 'bit of what he fancies' that bothered me so much. I used to pretend to myself that my ire was the reasonable, measured reaction of someone who knows perfectly well no one should be eating a whole packet of bacon, never mind two, in one day; that it was the normal revulsion anyone would experience at this wanton gorging. But I've finally had to admit that what really drives me to distraction is the fact that he *can* eat all that. If he wants it he just has it. It's the fact that he is so relaxed about food and, on top of that, capable of burning off any physical signs of having wolfed down two packets of bacon, three eggs, and the rest in one sitting.

I mind because he can eat without a second thought, because it's nothing to him, because, for him and all others without 'issues', there is absolutely no emotional cost involved in the transaction. For him there's no agony, no tortured thinking about the feast for hours in advance, no hasty calorie counting, no wondering whether he deserves it, whether he's earned it. There's no weighing up how he'll feel after the meal, no contemplating whether, afterwards, he'll be plunged into a slurry of self-loathing, asking himself if it was all worth it now that there's nothing to look forward to and only that bloated feeling left to keep him company. In fact, for him, there's no thinking about it at all. It's an entirely pure exchange between him, the chicken, the pig, and a piece of porcelain the size of a manhole cover. As it should be, it's a turmoil-free, wholly pleasurable experience.

Whereas for me, even though I'm not *that* fat, the over-whelming effort required to not be ten times bigger is a daily – no, hourly – battle. I hate the fact that I can't saunter into the kitchen and make myself a huge fry-up. True, I rarely want one, but the fact that it's off limits even if I did fancy it annoys me intensely. Of course, it isn't, in absolute terms, off limits. Nothing is. If I want a fry-up I can have one. I'm not an idiot. But I'm nowhere close to being able just to have what I want and leave it at that. If I were, I'd probably be thin.

Susie Orbach wrote a short book called *On Eating* in which she gives some advice that is essentially sound but, in this context, frankly silly. 'If you want the chocolate biscuit,' she writes (I'm paraphrasing), 'have it. And if you want another, have that one too. Just think about each one, and whether you really want it, before you put it in your mouth.' Erm, hold on a minute . . . It's not really that simple a process. She might as well tell an alcoholic to go ahead and have that nip of whisky, and then another, and another, but only if they *really* feel like it. That's not how over-indulgence works. And it's certainly not how overindulgers operate.

If those of us who overeat, for whatever reason, were capable of summoning up the ability to consider each biscuit on its individual merits before consuming it, we'd hardly be likely to be the sort of person who overate in the first place. It's all very well telling someone to separate out self-loathing and bingeing from real desire, but you have to acknowledge it's a long and difficult process in which no diet, no self-help book, is going to work instant magic. It is never about pulling your socks up and not 'letting yourself go'. It's about changing the attitude of a lifetime – and that takes time, no matter what glossy magazines tell us.

If I hadn't, like most Western women, experienced a lifetime of being told by parents, advertisers, employers, the media, etc., that my weight and looks were inexorably linked to how worthy a person I was, to how much I had to offer the world, to how I'd be judged as a person, then of course I'd bloody well be able to stand coolly over a tin of chocolate digestives assessing exactly how many I wanted with my cup of tea. Leaving aside for a moment the fact that my particular neurotic make-up informs my wrestling match with every single 'naughty' item that ever passes my lips, it's more generally relevant to point out that taste, enjoyment, and – hey, dare I say it? – greed also make up some of the moves in this hugely complicated cha-cha-cha.

It would appear that I just can't get used to men's 'entitlement' to eat whatever they want. I'm constantly railing against the difference between male and female metabolisms and the injustice of it all. It's no good blaming it on nature, as if that'd make one gaily feel better about it. It's not fair; and to make matters worse it's not as if the social pressure on men to be slim and good-looking is equal to that put on women.

And as if all that isn't bad enough, when men do eventually put on weight (as they tend to) later in life, they don't then think it reflects badly on them as people, or that it diminishes their chances of success in any field, personal or professional, or that they're less attractive (what an idea . . .). They just think they've acquired a beer gut, no more, no less!

The mother of all diets

As an adult, even before I had children, I found it hard enough to diet. That is to say, I didn't. I mean I did, of course I did. I dieted plenty of times.

And sometimes I succeeded – that is if by 'success' we mean I lost a few pounds. But I put them back on again so, you know, that's not really success, is it? It was always, always, always a fierce struggle to eat less, as I trudged along towards what I imagined would be a Better Me.

So carefree eating isn't something of which I've had much experience (have any women?). And dieting successfully is not, whatever anyone will have you believe, straightforward. Dieting requires you to adhere to an unwritten contract with yourself. (The contract specifies that you hereby agree to reduce what you eat FOR A VERY LONG TIME, if not, in fact, THE REST OF YOUR LIFE. And who precisely is going to sue you if you happen to break a contract with yourself?)

How that plays out, practically, is that every single time you respond to your hunger, or prepare something to eat, or are invited out to eat, you must be on high alert, poised to pounce on any and all rogue temptations, any normal attraction to anything remotely tempting, tasty, or delicious. Without any training, armed only with the hard-to-hold-on-to notion that thin equals better, you have to teach yourself how to nip in the bud all subconscious and instant reactions to food.

It's as though you're your own police force *and* the lawbreaker at the same time. If a water company provides water to your home, they undertake to maintain the pipes delivering the water, set a price for this service, and employ people to provide it. They aren't also charged with monitoring the consistent quality and execution of that service – that job falls to Ofwat whose byline is 'protecting consumers, promoting value, and safeguarding the future'. Going on a diet means you have to become your own regulatory body – a one-person Off-fat.

Good God, dieting would be a doddle if someone else were running your Off-fat for you – 'protecting consumers' (that'd be you), 'promoting value' (helping you maintain 'thin' in your sights), and 'safeguarding the future' (i.e. stopping you from putting the weight back on). Hey, that must be what it's like being a married man on a diet. All the men I know who've managed to lose weight have done so with the help of their wives, who do the shopping and cooking for them (as with my journalist friend who oh-so-helpfully recommended his diet to me). No wonder they dropped a few pounds: they've got their own personal Off-fat right there at home. Well, hello?! Where's my Off-fat?

For most women hoping to lose weight there's no such luck. Unless you can afford a cook, a trainer, and a nutritionist *and* are prepared to eat either alone or separated from friends and family, you're on your own on this statistically hopeless quest for thinness. This is even truer for women with children. A cohabiting woman with kids who's trying to lose weight is running not only Off-fat but Off-ensure-kids-and-partner-get-fed, too.

And diets have a 95 per cent failure rate. Ninety-five per cent! Research shows not only that diets fail but that the vast majority of dieters regain *more* weight than they lost by dieting in the first place. Most people's body weight and shape do *not* change dramatically within their adult lifetime unless subjected to radical changes in lifestyle and exercise habits. Taking these facts on board, how could the added complication of being responsible for feeding *other* people as well feel like anything other than yet another obstacle towards winning the war on fat? Kids are growing all the time; they can and should consume a whole variety of things, many of which are positively at odds with a weight-loss regime. In fact, a lot of the stuff my kids eat would make me fatter if I so much as looked at it.

Providing food for other people who are unable to provide for themselves sometimes feels like being one of those hamsters on a relentlessly spinning wheel: there's no prospect of it ever ending. Every time I return from the shops with yet more provisions I feel as though I've just pushed a very heavy ball up a very steep hill, and immediate consumption of those provisions makes me feel as if the ball and I have careered right back down the hill, only to have to start the whole journey again. Feeding children is unremitting, it's rarely fun, and even more rarely appreciated – and why should it be? You're their mum, and that's what mums (and a few dads) do. (My mum, of course, being the exception.)

And I *want* my kids to expect to be fed. I don't want them to wonder if there'll be any supper, as we did at our house when we were kids. I want them to grow up feeling the security and love that plentiful, nourishing food offers. I'd give anything for my children to have a healthy, non-combative relationship with food, but, ye gods and little fishes, being responsible for ensuring that happens while also attempting to be a fascinating person *and* trying to lose weight is nigh on impossible. Here I am, on a daily basis, trying to dream up new and exciting ways to 'present' a green vegetable and yet being held at figurative gunpoint by the packet of biscuits my husband bought and casually popped in the cupboard 'for later'. I've been incapable of not thinking about them since the moment they took up residence. How on earth can a mother be expected to invent a way to render broccoli alluring while under siege from a milk chocolate digestive?

Meanwhile, further complicating my responsibility to feed the whole family is my default position that I don't need to eat regularly. Why would I need to eat? I'm fat, and fat people don't need to eat. We've eaten enough already;

look at us. I do, however, know that the kids need to eat, so I'll find myself alone in the house with their food, but nothing for me to eat. I can eat their leftovers once they've definitely been Left Over, but I can't 'take food from their mouths' by including myself among those who qualify for the nice food in the first place. They deserve food; I don't. Obviously, I can't eat their stuff – but I *can* eat something bought for them but subsequently rejected, because that falls into the category of 'unwanted food', and that's OK to eat because by eating that I'm not 'letting food go to waste'. So I will eat one of the 36 chewy bars they said they liked and then changed their minds about, but only after I'd bought a mountain of the wretched things on a BOGOF offer.

As it happens I don't like them, either – they claim to be 'apricot' but the taste is alarmingly reminiscent of one of those naff scented sticks you put in a lav to 'disguise' the smell of poo. It's like eating something made by Glade. Does that stop me? No, of course not. My reaction, of course, is: look, let's face it, they're there, they are paid for (by me, to boot), and apart from the small matter of tasting completely and utterly revolting, there's nothing actually, technically wrong with them. Who better to finish off these inedible snack bars than me, since I don't deserve nice food chosen by me to provide myself with tasty nourishment? I simply can't buy appealing food specifically for myself. I can eat if what I'm eating is horrible, or left over (naturally), or just 'there', but no thought, preparation, or expectation must go into supplying myself with good, tasty food because that would mean I thought I deserved it. And thinking

I deserved something nice would be a slippery slope: next I'd be eating whatever I liked because it tasted nice, and then where would I be?

If you're not blessed with it already, there's no time or space to develop an enjoyment of food when you're feeding children – there's a bloody assault course to be conquered every single day. And now there's the whole five-a-day thing to be achieved, too. And that's five *different*, if you please, fruits and veg. Don't go thinking you can get away with two apples as part of the five – oh no, they must be different, got it? And then research indicates that kids should also have a green vegetable every day. Hah! Good luck with that, particularly when green vegetables are, as if by magic, the very things most kids can suddenly find they have a new, 'real' (exclusively to them, natch) reason not to eat the moment one sails into view. And everything's got to be steamed, not boiled, so, while you're juggling the plates, don't forget that, either.

So, as mothers, we are charged not only with preparing and providing the meals every day but also with ensuring that all government guidelines are adhered to. A tall order – on top of which, we have to *not* eat their leftovers (even though they're delicious, right there, and surely better eaten than binned?) *and* help them form a healthily unfrantic attitude to things like chocolate biscuits. It's a minefield littered with hidden bombs for someone who has an un-relaxed relationship with food in general, and a positively aggressive one with sweets, cakes, and biscuits.

I washed some grapes today. (It's not something I do routinely, I must confess. I'm not a great believer in washing fruit. I mean, if it's sprayed with stuff that can kill things then it's hardly likely to come off with a quick rinse, is it?) Anyway, as I shook them dry I remembered my mother telling us not to eat the grapes in the fruit bowl. 'Who are they for, then?' I'd ask. 'I don't know, but not you,' Mum would reply. 'They're too expensive for you.' That is as true today as it was 35 years ago: grapes are expensive compared to other fruits. However, Mum's reasoning had nothing to do with saving the grapes for more deserving people and everything to do with just 'saving' the grapes, letting the grapes be in the house for longer than they would be if her kids simply ate them the moment they laid eyes on them. Of course, this often meant the grapes would go mouldy before they ever got eaten but, for my mother, this meant that at least they'd *been* there for a while. She'd got value for money. The expensive grapes had earned their keep, justifying the hefty expenditure by gracing the fruit bowl with their presence for more than the measly half an hour they would have got if I'd eaten them. Mum had not shelled out a few pounds for fruit only to have it disappear the second it was through the front door.

And now that I'm a mother I understand how she felt. Feeding a family can feel like trying to fill a bath with a coffee spoon and with the plug out. My husband, predictably enough, doesn't understand this feeling at all. Why would he? He's male and he doesn't have an elaborate exchange with eating. When he was growing up he was given food regularly (by his mother, i.e. a woman) with no attendant discussions about his size or his need for it. It was there on demand.

So, with a certain amount of nervousness and steeling myself not to say 'not too many', I let my kids have biscuits, chocolate, and crisps, and so far they haven't tried to stuff down an entire cake whilst hiding in a cupboard – I don't think, anyway. However, they're only young and as yet I haven't taken a theatrically loud sharp intake of breath or rolled my eyes wearily when they reach for a 'treat'. Maybe it'll be harder when or if one of them starts to get plump but continues to eat as if they weren't, eat as if they were as slim as they were before, eat as their un-plump siblings and friends do – good God, what then?

Feeding Mum

Thanks to a range of experiences provided by life and many entertainers, most notably Elton John and Shakespeare, all of us know that our existence ends, and very often does so in a remarkably similar way to how it started.

We're all aware that as elderly people approach the end of their lives they often have the same needs as babies – to be cleaned, fed, washed, and looked after as if they were infants. Difficult and distasteful as these tasks may be to undertake, particularly when for our own parents, we engage in completing this aspect of the 'circle of life' because years earlier they've taken care of us in the same way. Now it's payback time.

And so it was with my mother. But, as you now know, feeding me when I was little wasn't ever high on Mum's list of Things to Do. Yet, strangely, in the end I fed her. And although I was very happy to do it, the irony didn't escape me. Food, yet again, played a big, last part in my relationship with Mum.

Around mid-March 2009, early one evening, Mum rang to tell me she'd been sick immediately after eating.

'What did you eat, Mum?' I asked, not unkindly, but in a brisk tone by now familiar to us both. She knew it suggested that whatever she'd eaten was very likely to have been old, mouldy, or just plain off.

She laughed. 'Yes, well, it was some lentils that have been sitting in the pan for a few days now – probably past their best.'

I laughed. In defiant reaction to her austere Scottish childhood of open windows and cold bathwater, Mum now kept her house incredibly warm, and the tropical temperature meant that any food kept out of the fridge turned bad almost immediately.

This time, though, she went on, slightly tentatively: 'But I didn't feel at all ill. It just came straight up without any warning.'

That did sound a bit odd, and I was a little more concerned – but not greatly worried. We agreed that we'd speak the next day and see how she felt then.

But she was sick again the next day, and the next, and the next. Eventually, she was being sick every time she ate. We talked to her doctor, who decided that Mum needed a proper check-up.

She was admitted to hospital and given a lovely room of her own with a view right over London. There, she was as happy as a kid in a toy shop. She returned to her usual robust, intellectually lively self, revelling in the gentle, efficient care provided by the array of mumsy, chatty nurses. Over several weeks of numerous and sometimes invasive tests, it became clear that locating exactly what was wrong with Mum was going to take time. Meanwhile, the doctors urged us to ensure that she ate regular meals, for which she had no appetite at all.

So, every time I visited her, practically every day, we'd end up squabbling over her food. By a quirk of fate I was now spoon-feeding, literally, my own mother. She was more than capable, both physically and mentally, of feeding herself, but said she preferred me to do it. So I'd sit and babble away, trying to distract her from the main aim of getting at least something, however little, inside her – just as you do with a kid. Thankfully, I didn't have to resort to making choo-choo sounds or pretending the forkful was a train going into a tunnel. Mum was ill, not demented. Apart from a bit of the occasional school-dinner type of squishy pudding, which she loved, Mum really didn't fancy eating at all and wasn't even hungry. She knew she had to eat something to stay alive, if nothing else. Nonetheless, entirely typically, she put up all possible resistance. So every day we'd go through the ritual: me, sitting on the side of her bed, a laden fork in my hand, trying to tempt her with a bit of food, while she complained, groaned, or, if she was in a bad mood, effed and blinded and told me to stop annoying her, how tedious I was with my constant nagging, how boring I could be . . .

Of course she didn't really want me to stop. She liked the attention. One of the things it took me years, if not a lifetime, to learn about my mother was that she craved attention but didn't always know how to seek it positively. So, if she got your attention by annoying you, so be it; the end result, for her, justified the means. And since she was always relentlessly unapologetic, she didn't stop herself when she realised you were getting into a bate: she was just pleased she'd got a rise out of you and therefore the attention she sought. I didn't get cross with her in the hospital, though. The situation seemed too serious for that.

And our little routine ended up being quite a laugh. She'd roll her eyes, exhale flamboyantly, slump her shoulders, and slither down into her bed every time the lunch trolley hove into view. While I took the tray from the nurse, Mum would go through an extravagant series of facial grimaces, trying to mime to me that the 'wretched tray' was not to be left because she wasn't going to eat anything on it, even though she'd knew I'd take it. I'd plop the tray over Mum's legs, load up the fork, and round and round we'd go, day after day – her refusing the food, and me cajoling her.

One day, out of the blue, Mum said, 'That's why I didn't eat when I was young. Because when I didn't, my mother would come and sit with me and feed me. That was the only time she ever spent alone with me and I liked it.'

Although I knew my mother felt she'd been badly neglected by her own mother, and there was compelling evidence to support her belief that this was the case, I'd never heard this particular story. I asked her to tell it to me. It turned out that, as part of their efforts to ensure their only child wasn't spoilt and – wait for it – didn't think she was 'special', Mum's parents decided they should treat her exactly as they did all the boys, the pupils at the school they ran. Consequently, from the age of four, Mum slept in the school dormitory and ate all her meals in the school refectory, even though, unlike the boys, her parents lived right there, in a house on the grounds. It's easy to understand why Mum seized on this means of securing time alone with her mother and getting the individual attention she obviously craved – any child would. Mum told me that, on these occasions, the refectory would slowly empty as the boys made their way back to their classes or to bed, while her mother sat patiently with her, making sure that she finished her meal. If those were the only times Mum felt she had her mother's attention, it's no wonder that food became so steeped in meaning for her.

When it finally became clear that Mum was very ill – in fact, that this was the end – she bore the news with astonishing courage and equanimity. In stark contrast to the childish, petulant, melodramatic person she could often be, she was accepting, dignified, and adult about the news, saying, in a completely matter-of-fact tone, 'Well, everyone has to die sometime and I've had a good life. I'm ready to go.' Not once did she express rage or disappointment, and she left her loved ones peacefully. (Mum did, in fact, have a very good life, after we'd grown up and she reformed a friendship with Dad – not because of those two facts but because, as she once said, 'I don't think I knew what I thought or felt about anything until after I was 60.' As she'd got older she became more able to appreciate stuff. However, she remained pretty combative right to the last.)

While there are many things I strive to do differently from my mother in relation to my kids, I would like to think that at the very end I'll be able to leave them with as much grace and acceptance of the inevitable as Mum did her children.

Dieting makes you fat

The trouble with eating is that you have to do it. You won't stay alive if you don't eat. At all. You will stay alive if you stop drinking too much alcohol. You'll also continue to live if you stop smoking. But you won't if you stop eating. Dieting requires you to continue to eat – but just less. To diet you have to stop eating a bit. You try recommending to a chronic smoker or alcoholic that they carry on with their habit but just dial it down a bit. What's more, smokers and drinkers feel better when they stop. But who feels good when they're hungry? When has hunger ever helped? Unless you're very ill, it doesn't make you feel good. It's not like a gruelling exercise regime, which is mighty tedious but feels good after you've done it and helps you stave off death (so they say, anyway). Helping an old lady with her shopping is boring, but gives the old lady a hand and makes you feel like a good person. Good God, giving your partner a blow-job isn't much fun but it sure gives a great deal of pleasure, so there's at least some 'good' in it. Hunger doesn't promote any 'good' whatsoever. It only leads to being hungrier. It becomes an all-consuming obsession. Never mind Kingsley Amis's claim that 'being born with a penis is like being handcuffed to a maniac for life'. From what I've heard, a penis in repose is no bother at all; and, when it is standing to attention, its needs can be dispatched pretty swiftly by its owner, should no one else be around to oblige.

Dieting is a see-saw between spells of reduced consumption spurred on by self-loathing, and diet-wrecking flashes of self-esteem. To diet successfully you need to *not* like yourself, a great deal, *all the time*. Every time a piece of chocolate cake hoves into view or a crisp packet rustles invitingly, the wannabe thinny has to be alert, ready to pounce on the fatty who yearns to tuck in.

I used to diet; in fact, more of my life has been spent on a diet than not on a diet. Who knows what I'd look like if I'd never started dieting? I'd start diet after diet after diet, each taken from a newly purchased, newly launched-as-'the one' diet book. Like everyone else who supports the hugely profitable diet industry, I imagined that each time was going to be 'it'. I'd definitely be able to stick to this one and then I'd be thin. It was a bit like marrying Elizabeth Taylor: everyone goes in thinking, With me, it's going to work. And friends, keen to see a new me, gave me helpful hints to spur me on, such as putting an unflattering picture of myself up on the fridge door or buying an outfit a couple of sizes too small, or skipping one meal a day entirely.

The F-Plan, the Cabbage Soup, the All-Eggs, the

Grapefruit, the Hay, the Scarsdale, the All-Protein, the 10-lbs-in-Ten-Days, the Miracle, the Ultimate, the G-I, the Blood Group, the Thin-Thighs-in-Thirty-Days, the Never-Eat-in-the-Nude (OK, I made that one up, but it works, doesn't it, because you don't, do you?) – every single useless, preposterously unmanageable diet ever invented, I tried them all, clinging desperately to each one as it appeared, praying that this would be the life raft that would carry me off to that paradise, a new and better me. Of course, apart from no permanent poundage loss, many of those diets had side effects you were 'warned' about but completely ignored in your frenzy to get thin. Thanks to some of those regimes, in my time, I have let out enough wind to power a hot-air balloon across the Channel, had breath so bad it would have embarrassed a moose, and been so constipated I contemplated using a dessertspoon to relieve the discomfort.

And I see there's a new diet 'weight-loss programme' on the market. It's called Celebrity Slim. Talk about 'does what it says on the tin'. Forget about an unflattering photo of yourself or a dress two sizes too small. Why not have a celebrity's figure in your sights as your incentive? Not a specific celebrity, mind you: the word 'celebrity' is used to conjure up everything you surely want as motivation. It's not called that because a celebrity invented it. It's not even endorsed by a celebrity. It is called that, presumably, because everyone wants to be slim like a celebrity. So blindingly obvious is the aspiration the product name is trying to encourage they might as well have called it Beckham Slim,

Hilton Slim, or Cole Slim – actually no, that last one sounds like a salad, and you wouldn't want to evoke something to eat, would you?

Anyway, most celebrities eat only just enough to stay alive. Naomi Campbell announced the other day that she kept in shape by drinking a shake made up of water, maple syrup, lemon juice, and cayenne pepper and nothing else at all for usually 'around 18 days'. Nothing else. Apparently Gwyneth Paltrow and Beyoncé also use this system for, erm, maintaining existence. I don't mind what they do: it's the use of these completely unfeasible methods for 'keeping in shape' as a stick to beat the rest of us with to which I object. Since it's apparently doable by them and they're only human, the reports imply, it's doable by us. There's no mention of hugely differing lifestyles, income, and access to the wide range of opportunities that make taking on a liquid-only regime a possibility.

Never mind the bonkers mantra 'nothing tastes as good as skinny feels' – that lot has obviously never tasted the perfect bread-and-butter pudding. Forget dieting: it doesn't work. Our time and energy would be much better spent learning how to trust our own instincts, how to recognise them, and how to validate them. That's a tall order, though, in a world that is constantly overwhelming us, particularly women, with the message 'be like this – not like that'.

Dieting is phenomenally hard – impossible in my case. Yet it isn't as hard as accepting that there is no miracle diet, no food combination, no low-GI regime, no discovery of intolerances which if stuck to will be *the* key to unlocking the door to weight loss. The hardest thing of all to accept is that it's just maths: you lose weight if you eat less. I'm finally there – and it's just that I want the cake more than I want to be thin.

Not eating, just neatening

The road to hell is paved with good intentions. For example, I have a small pair of dumbbells sitting in my kitchen, on the counter, in view but not in the way. They've been there for, oooh, about three and half years. They're there because that's where they landed up after I'd bought them – you know, carefully placed so that I'd see them every day and thereby be reminded to do arm exercises to rid myself of those horrible flappy arm undercarriages.

I've never once touched them. I tell a lie: I had to move them to get to something they were blocking. Other than that, they've sat there since the day they were bought. I'm not, however, going to get rid of them, because that would mean admitting they were completely redundant. One day, very soon, I'll be needing them for those exercises, OK? So there they'll remain for another few years, gathering dust until, erm, well, until . . . I don't know, actually. Maybe until I admit that the 'bingo wings' are a fact of life and here to stay; that I am going to have those flappy bits until I die.

My house is littered with untouched fat-reducing props that were the very thing, each one of them, that was going to spur me into taking up a hitherto unfamiliar exercise. They were going to work because they were new and, well, just there every day, acting as a reminder to do whatever exercise they aided. Who doesn't know someone who bought an exercise bike that now acts as a clothes horse but that they won't or can't get rid of because one day, soon, they're going to get fit?

Oh, the tricks we use to delude ourselves! For example, picking at food when standing up and not using a plate, because that way it doesn't count – that's the main trick of which I'm guilty. I don't accept that I'm eating because I don't *acknowledge* that I'm eating. The food isn't laid out on a plate, nicely prepared for a person who's taken a decision to eat it. Therefore I think you'll find that I'm not, in fact, eating it. QED.

Here's a little scene that occurred earlier today. I'm standing at the kitchen counter. I'm eating a second hot cross bun. I don't really want it. (Not, remember, that I'm generally able to discern the difference between when I do and don't want food, but I'm pretty confident that this time I don't want it.) I've already had one and it was really nice – soft, sweet, and fruity – so now I'm trying to replicate the sensation it gave me when I ate it by having another. I know it's one too many, but I can't stop now. I also know I'll feel really bad when I've eaten it, but *while* I'm eating it feels good and tastes gorgeous.

I've eaten it now. I feel too full, so that's not great. Why didn't I just have one? I know why. Well, seeing as

I 'shouldn't' have been having even one in the first place, why not be extra disgusting and self-indulgent and have two? In fact, you might say it's a major personal achievement that I didn't eat all four. Yet I derive no pride or satisfaction from *not* having eaten the whole packet. Two is ample to make me feel bad about myself. Feeling bad about what I've eaten, or even about having eaten anything at all, is a familiar sensation. It's what I feel every time I eat anything nice.

Later the same day. The kids have just come home from school. Once they've rejected my kisses and groaned theatrically at commands that they change out of their uniforms, read improving books, and practise their times tables, I open their lunchboxes. Each contains more than half the remains of a perfectly good tuna, sweetcorn, and mayo (light, natch) brown-bread sandwich. 'Anything wrong with your sandwiches, kids?' I ask, adopting an unconcerned, no-pressure-just-enquiring-it-really-couldn't-matter-less, faux-cheery tone of voice. 'Nah, it was fine, just didn't fancy all of it,' they reply, almost in unison. That's great, fantastic even. Just as it should be. This is the perfect attitude for them to have. Good for them: they didn't fancy the whole sandwich so they didn't eat it. Brilliant. I should be proud of myself for having cultivated in my kids such a relaxed and healthy attitude to food. They've shown an admirable lack of guilt and absolutely no hint of greed. They ate half and left the rest because, quite simply, they did not feel the need to eat the whole thing. What could be more balanced?

However, that is them and, sadly, still very much not me. So, faced with two halves of uneaten sandwiches, what do I do? Eat them. Of course I do. I eat every last morsel of both discarded lunches, including the crumbs of their snack bars. And I don't want any of it. I'm not the least bit hungry (I've already had those hot cross buns, not to mention lunch), but there it all is, taunting me, and what's more, there is absolutely nothing wrong with it – for the love of God, none of it's even off! On top of all that, *I* made them. I got up 20 minutes early to bloody well make them. Existentially, it *is* quite annoying that they got rejected.

I'm not annoyed with the kids, though. I'm annoyed with the sandwiches. I don't want them to come home and make me eat them. I want them not to be here at all. I don't want to be faced with the choice. Choice? Hah! There is no choice. Discarded food in my house, no matter how unappealing, must be eaten and, if I'm the only one who will eat it, then so be it. In fact, discarded food anywhere is in danger of being hoovered up by me. You see, in that moment I'm not eating, oh no: I am neatening. What I'm actually doing is clearing up. It's more of a public service than a sign of a dysfunctional tug-of-war with leftovers. I realise that sounds like the most extraordinary self-delusion, but that is how the thinking goes.

It's the same process when eating out with a pal. I don't order my companion's chips; granted, I might have encouraged them to order some, but they ordered them, not me. And they are just there on the table and, like as not, unfinished. (You see, if my pal is the sort of person who orders chips in the first place, then they're also very likely to be the sort of person who doesn't finish them off. Annoying, isn't it?) The chips have been discarded and are about to 'go to waste', and obviously I can't let that happen. But I only ever eat something someone else has ordered off their plate. That way I don't have to address the thought that I might actually want whatever it is they've ordered. *They* ordered it; it's on *their* plate; so I'm not actually eating it.

And food cannot be wasted, even if the cost is that I, in a gesture of heroic self-sacrifice, get fatter. Anybody brought up in the UK after the Second World War is familiar with the notion that not wasting food is much better than throwing it away for no better reason than because no one fancies it. But a vast chasm now lies between people who've managed to stop bringing to mind that guilt-inducing parental nag every time they so much as consider chucking out food and those of us who've woven it tightly into the tapestry that makes up our relationship with food.

It's not logical, of course, to hold that it is 'better' to eat bits of unwanted food than to throw them away. That chucked-away food isn't any more likely to find its way from your stomach to the starving in Africa than it is to get there from the bottom of the bin. But it *feels* a little less like wanton waste when food is eaten than it does when it's tipped into a black plastic bag.

After all, getting fucked up about food isn't logical. It takes years and years to get really fucked up, and you have to start early, when you're a kid, to be really good at it. All the delusional not-ordering-chips, not-on-a-plate stuff just happens automatically by the time you're grown-up. And not eating, just neatening, happens automatically. It happens when you're not officially eating, when you're doing something else, so you don't have to think about whatever it was you ate. You'll just have popped it into your mouth while you got on with emptying the lunchbox, wiping down the counter, making supper, asking about homework, wondering if you can squeeze a bit more work in after the kids have gone to bed, or just have a glass of wine.

The opportunities to engage in this kind of eating-on-autopilot present themselves a million times a day, and in particular to women with children. Sure, nowadays we're all being invited to imagine ourselves as girlies frolicking merrily in front of an overpriced cooker, tossing off delectable dishes in a matter of minutes with a cheery smile. But it's all bollocks. All those books, TV programmes, and related products really do is make women feel inadequate: inadequate that they don't put enough work into being perfect for their spouses and their offspring; inadequate that they aren't running a successful business at the same time as making oversized cupcakes; inadequate that they haven't yet created a range of 'fun' kidswear/kitchenware/furniture/corporate nicknacks, when apparently all it takes to achieve all of this and so much more is the ability to cock a leg in a flirty fashion while standing in front of a £4,000 Aga.

Another key element to deluding yourself when eating is free food. Free food isn't fattening. For food to qualify as 'free' you have to have not ordered it, not cooked it, not in any way gone through the process of acquiring or preparing it and best of all not paid for it. It's just somehow magically there. You haven't had to think about whether it's OK to have the offending item, whether you're thin enough, or on a diet currently, or suddenly the sort of person who casually

213

orders stuff like chips and puddings. You simply don't need to deal with any of that baggage because someone else is holding it, and you're only having a bite anyway. How could it hurt?! If it were possible to section off my 'fat bits' and trace back exactly what was responsible for each and every pound of flesh, then I think I'd find that my bum was entirely made up of a lifetime's 'Can I just have a taste?'

If your earliest memories of eating and food in general were filled with warnings that certain foods were naughty, off limits, special treats, and all the other emotive labels given to 'fattening' food, then they're bound to take on a power way out of kilter with their actual capacity to turn you into a fattie. If, added to that, you were told these items pose particular danger to you, as someone biologically prone to weight gain, and threaten to stop you being everything you might otherwise be, then you're likely to have had bad eating habits from the very start. For how do you ever develop a balanced enjoyment of something if you're never allowed to even sample it in the first place?

Wrong thinking

One of my closest friends is a woman called Helen. She's nine years older than me and in many ways she's been more than a friend: ever since we met 35 years ago, she's been a mentor to me, too. We have very different approaches to life but a shared sense of humour and very similar levels of self-esteem, oscillating unpredictably, for both of us, between illogically low and ludicrously high.

Helen has always been thin but has always thought she's fat. She now cringes with shame when I remind her of the times – I was in my late teens and she in her mid-twenties – when she used to say to me every single day, in person or on the phone, 'You know, if you lost weight you'd be a "*Thanks*, God …" girl.' A '*Thanks*, God …' girl was the nickname she gave to girls who were pretty *and* slim *and* clever – a sarcastically expressed faux gratitude to the Almighty for creating a girl who was everything every other girl would want to be. Of course, she meant it as an encouragement and a compliment. All I needed to qualify for the title was to lose weight since, according to her, I already had two out of the three boxes ticked.

I never made the cut. We laugh about it now, and Helen says, 'I don't know what I was thinking, but that's what I believed then. Blame my mother.' Her mother, despite being a successful and intelligent career woman who was happily married to Helen's father for life, had taught her daughter that men leave women who 'let themselves go', and what's more without a backward glance. Helen grew up – as many, many girls still do today – being fed the message that a man's loyalty and emotional attachment to his partner will rank (if at all) way below his interest in her physical appeal. And, almost worse than that depressing message, if she does 'let herself go' he can't be held responsible for the inevitable consequences.

As a theory, a belief, a code of practice, a law for life, it sounds completely implausible and positively comic. And there are, of course, heaps of men more emotionally advanced than that doctrine suggests. But challenging these beliefs is not so much to do with finding data to prove incontrovertibly that x many men left their partner because she'd got fat versus y many men who stayed *even though* she'd got fat. It's all to do with how women see themselves portrayed in the wider world and how and what they learn to value in themselves as a result.

To this day, if you use the media as your guide, it appears that there's no worse way for a woman to be than to 'let herself go' and put on weight, or not to lose it quickly following childbirth, or just to be overweight and not care about it. One way or another, women must pay for 'allowing' themselves to be physically unappealing – and what's more unappealing than to be overweight? The cost of 'payment' ranges hugely: some of us succumb to eating disorders, some get sucked into the toxic mixture of envy, sneering, and self-loathing peddled by the celebrity magazines every week and some spend a lifetime supporting the diet industry's massive profits, to name but a few.

Most women in the UK wear a size 14 or 16. Most women think they'd look (feel, *be*) better if they lost half a stone or so. Most women think they're fat. My stepmother, Hilary, was the skinniest person you could ever wish to meet, in fact, very often too skinny. She had a very good degree from Oxford, a successful career and marriage, two lovely sons – all the things that are supposed to make you feel fulfilled and happy – yet all her life she thought she was fat. My friend Kathy, a cancer research scientist in a very rare and important field, probably wears a size 14, if that; she thinks she's fat. Another friend, another Helen, a writer and a medieval historian, is a slim size 10; she thinks she's fat. I can't think of a female friend who doesn't think she ought to lose some weight. From where I stand, most women, irrespective of their achievements, seem to think they're fat, or at the very least that they fail to measure up in some way to a fantasy ideal that they believe is not a fantasy but actually an ideal achievable if only they tried hard enough.

Why do we do this? Moreover, why do we let others tell us this is the case? We already have proof that shit, sometimes awful shit, happens not just to us but to thin (and pretty, rich, and famous) people as well. We know that their extra qualifications, their sacrifices at the altar of thinness, didn't earn them immunity. Why do we allow ourselves to believe being thin is the Holy Grail? Why do we revere women, and a tiny minority at that, who *aren't* like us? What's wrong with admiring women who *are* like us – isn't that good enough? Why should we beat ourselves up for not being perfect? Who, after all, is 'perfect', and, as shit happens to them, too, how exactly is their life better protected from knocks? Whose definition of perfect will we accept and how will we know when we've got there?

Women have plenty of evidence to support the fear that to keep a man's love they must never take their eye off the ball. Take the dismal way in which the woe-filled stories of Cheryl Cole, Victoria Beckham, and Tess Daly are reported. Though the tone might imply that the woman has been 'wronged', the underlying (but, hey, usually overt) message is always, 'Well, she was away/working/fat/pregnant – she wasn't watching his every move, so of course he got bored, lonely, and wasn't getting sex. What does she expect?'

I once went to several Paris fashion shows as the guest of a pal who built sets for the catwalk. The models were so thin – bones sticking out everywhere – it brought tears to my eyes. No one else seemed to mind, or even notice. If this had been Crufts and the dogs were that emaciated, there'd have been a national outcry. No amount of dog breeders claiming that the dogs' outfits 'looked better like that' would have appeased the righteous anger sparked by the trainers' inhumanity. Yet, apart from the occasional and praiseworthy stand taken by a rare few, we don't seem to think that ill-looking girls being used to sell clothes to young women is that big a deal.

Every single one of us needs to reset our channels and stop agreeing to think of ourselves as too fat when we're not, or not worthy if we don't compare to models. I'm aware this is a bit rich coming from someone who's admitted she still wrangles with food and body image; but the fact remains that I know I do this and probably always will, and I'm making my dissent heard. I'm claiming my right to have a bit of cake irrespective of and in spite of how I 'ought' to look. I'm not pretending to be a Champion of Fat. I'm banging the drum for It's OK Not To Be Thin. This doesn't mean I'm recommending putting on five stone, unless that's what you fancy. It means I think we all need to learn to challenge every single message we get that tells us we ought to want to be different from how we are. I'm not advocating unhealthy eating, stuffing our faces with fast food, and lying in front of the TV all day long. Taking a stand against the tyranny of the myth that thin equals perfect does not mean that the opposite of thin is morbid obesity, slothfulness, and idleness. It means refusing to buy into the dogma that our worth is inevitably and permanently tied up to our size. It takes time, and (as I well know) a certain amount of grit, but, if we ordinary women, the vast majority, don't, then who will?

If I want to knock a story off the front page, I just change my hairstyle.

Hillary Clinton

Happy ending?

I've just been down to the kitchen. My computer, on which I write, is in a room that is also the spare bedroom at the top of the house. See? I can't even have a proper office. Having A Proper Office would mean I think I deserve one, that my career merits one. Hah! No, it's much better to have a crappy, wonky MDF table that cost £20 (bought at an Ikea sale, if you please, as if tables not on sale in Ikea aren't cheap enough) stuck into a recess in the spare room, because that way it's just sort-of there, and not really an office, not officially. And therefore, importantly, not inviting people to treat it as a proper office for producing proper things that earn money. No, that would seem much too much as if I expected to earn money by writing on my computer, in my office. And who on earth do I think I am, planning on earning money from writing, for goodness' sake? Writing is a proper job, not like acting which, after all, is just glorified mucking about. Let's face it, I'm not someone like Patricia Highsmith or Barbara Kingsolver – they are proper writers. I'm just someone who fell upon writing and got lucky.

I realise this mindset is still a bit bonkers at my age, but I'm just telling you what the voice of the little monster sitting on my shoulder says. I can hear him (I'm sure it's a male voice), but I've got better at not listening to him, not paying attention to what he's saying. He's been there all my life, remember, constantly reminding me that I'm not worthy. When I first started writing, my dad was obviously poleaxed with terror at the idea that a publisher had somehow mistaken me for someone who was capable of writing a book that anyone would be interested in buying. So he began to ring up with uncharacteristic frequency to tell me about various press mentions of books by my peers, and in particular Helen Fielding's forthcoming *Bridget Jones*, which he knew about because he read the paper in which the columns appeared.

'Don't you think it's a mistake to write a book like yours when she's writing that one?' was one of his best queries. I managed to summon up enough self-belief to respond with, 'Dad, would you like me to give the money back to the publishers?' 'Err, no, darling, but I think you should be forewarned.' When I asked how being forewarned would help, he didn't have an answer. I guess he couldn't bear the idea that I'd merrily trot into my publishers, proudly brandishing my finished book, not realising that I ought to be apologising for having dared to write one at the same time as, erm, someone else. His eventual defence was that he was trying to stop me 'getting ideas above my station'.

Anyway, back to where we were: now, today, both in actual fact and in terms of 'where I'm at' in my head pretty much all the time. It's lunchtime, we're in the kitchen, and I eat a pear. (Naturally, it's nearly off and covered with bruised brown bits; otherwise I'd have left it for the kids.) Then I eat a slice of cheese – actually two, but I'm kidding myself that it's one slice because they're both quite thin and I eat them on three oatcakes which are no one's idea of a treat, so they sort of excuse the cheese, as it were. Oh yes, and I have a bit of hummus, but there were signs of mould forming around the edge of the pot, so that's OK.

I consume the above standing and hanging up a wash in between mouthfuls, because I couldn't just eat at a table, off a plate. That would be like . . . well . . . like eating. Then I'd have to believe I was hungry enough to deserve the food and that my hunger was worth dirtying another plate for. (I've already worked out that after we've eaten tonight, assuming I do actually eat, then the dishwasher will be full enough to put on, whereas if I'd used a plate for lunch it would be too full to accommodate tonight's stuff, thereby maximising every possible opportunity not to sit down and eat lunch properly.) Hanging out the washing at the same time also means I wasn't really eating, and (even though I sort of was) I was using the time usefully, since eating is not useful or even necessary for me. And that was lunch.

So am I now a happy, slim person capable of eating what I want, when I want? Am I now capable of not eating too much when presented with a delicious array of foods?

Hah! I still finish off the kids' food, drink that last glass of wine when I know I've already had enough, go back to the buffet table at a party for another helping of whatever fantastic dish was on offer even though I've had ample ... and the rest. However, on the upside, I now fully accept that I was probably never going to be thin, unless I ate nothing at all, ever. And I accept that I actually don't want to be the woman who eats nothing because she believes her figure is more important than anything else about her. I accept that some of us were born to eat the same amount as others but 'show' it more. I accept that if you eat pudding you'll have a bigger arse than someone who never does. I accept that I'll never look great in jeans or strapless dresses or bikinis (oh God, what an idea!).

But I don't accept that I'm less of a person because I haven't denied myself the enjoyment of food. I don't and won't accept that women are still defined, above anything else, by how they look and how 'hard' they've worked to 'keep their figures'. I do a lot of exercise – yes, it's true, I run two or three miles four times a week. I'm pretty fit, but I drink and eat too and it would appear that that's the way the cookie crumbles (get it?). If my kids end up with a healthy attitude to food, if they eat what they want when they want, and if neither of them ever thinks a woman's size has anything to do with her popularity professionally, socially, or romantically, then I'll consider myself to have done a pretty good job. Currently, though, we're all battling against the mighty celebrity culture that encourages us *all* to prize famous women (and therefore ourselves) for their ability to starve themselves above all else.

But remember: there are many, many more of us than there are of them, so isn't this a battle we could win, if for no other reason than because, as we're so often told, we're worth it? Hah!

Acknowledgements

I would like, first and foremost, to acknowledge all my siblings, the three with whom I shared parents, if not parenting, Andrew, Matthew, and Christina, and the two with whom I shared a father, if not, perhaps, fathering, Alexander and Malcolm. No lawsuits, please.

I would also like to thank very much indeed my editor, Louise Haines, for her dogged pursuit, unswerving support, and truly unending patience. She's just the kind of editor someone with uneven self-esteem needs. The same goes for my agent, Sarah Lutyens, who really ought to have chucked me long ago. I owe a huge debt of gratitude, too, to my close friend Helen Castor without whom (I know everyone says this but in this case it's true) I could not have written this – so, all complaints to her.

Lastly, bucking the current trend, instead of a tattoo I'd just like to say in print, instead of on my back, Jeremy, Isabella, and Archie.